PROGRESS IN CLINICAL AND BIOLOGICAL RESEARCH

RECENT TITLES

Please contact the publisher for information about previous titles in this series.

Tumor Markers and Their Significance in the Management of Breast Cancer

Tumor Markers and Their Significance in the Management of Breast Cancer

Proceedings of a Workshop held in Bethesda, Maryland
March 6, 1985

Editors

Thomas Dao
Department of Breast Surgery
Roswell Park Memorial Institute
Buffalo, New York

Angela Brodie
Department of Pharmacology and
Experimental Therapeutics
University of Maryland School of Medicine
Baltimore, Maryland

Clement Ip
Organ Systems Coordinating Center
Roswell Park Memorial Institute
Buffalo, New York

ALAN R. LISS, INC. • NEW YORK

Address all Inquiries to the Publisher
Alan R. Liss, Inc., 41 East 11th Street, New York, NY 10003

Copyright © 1986 Alan R. Liss, Inc.

Printed in the United States of America

Library of Congress Cataloging-in-Publication Data
Main entry under title:

Tumor markers and their significance in the management
  of breast cancer.

  Sponsored by the Breast Cancer Working Group of the
Organ Systems Program, National Cancer Institute.
  Includes index.
    1. Breast—Cancer—Diagnosis—Congresses. 2. Tumor
markers—Congresses. 3. Tumor antigens—Congresses.
I. Ip, Clement. II. Dao, Thomas L. (Thomas Ling-Yuan),
1922-   . III. Brodie, Angela. IV. Organ Systems
Program (National Cancer Institute). Breast Cancer
Working Group. [DNLM: 1. Antigens, Neoplasms—analysis—
congresses. 2. Breast Neoplasms—diagnosis—congresses.
3. Neoplasms Proteins—analysis—congresses.
W1 PR668E v.204/WP 870 T925 1985]
RC280.B8T86 1986   616.99′449075   85-23902
ISBN 0-8451-5054-5

Contents

Contributors

H. Leon Bradlow, The Rockefeller University, 1230 York Avenue, New York, NY 10021 **[91]**

Francoise Capony, Unité d'Endocrinologie Cellulaire et Moléculaire (U 148), INSERM, 60, rue de Navacelles - 34100 Montpellier, France **[125]**

Roberto L. Ceriani, John Muir Cancer and Aging Research Institute, 2055 North Broadway, Walnut Creek, CA 94561 **[3]**

Mark W. Chandler, John Muir Cancer and Aging Research Institute, 2055 North Broadway, Walnut Creek, CA 94561 **[3]**

Thomas L. Dao, Department of Breast Surgery, Roswell Park Memorial Institute, 666 Elm Street, Buffalo, NY 14263 **[31]**

Parimal R. Desai, Department of Immunochemistry Research, Evanston Hospital, 2650 Ridge Avenue, Evanston, IL 60201 **[47]**

Lynn G. Dressler, Department of Medicine, University of Texas Health Sciences Center, 7703 Floyd Curl Drive, San Antonio, TX 78284 **[71]**

Dean P. Edwards, Department of Pathology, University of Colorado Health Sciences Center, 4200 East Ninth Avenue, Denver, CO 80262 **[71]**

Jack Fishman, The Rockefeller University, 1230 York Avenue, New York, NY 10021 **[91]**

Marcel Garcia, Unité d'Endocrinologie Cellulaire at Moléculaire (U 148), INSERM, 60, rue de Navacelles - 34100 Montpellier, France **[125]**

Fred J. Hendler, Department of Internal Medicine, The University of Texas Health Science Center, 5323 Harry Hines Blvd., Dallas, TX 75235 **[105]**

Richard J. Hershcopf, The Rockefeller University, 1230 York Avenue, New York, NY 10021 **[91]**

Diane House, Cancer Center, The University of Texas Health Science Center, 5323 Harry Hines Blvd., Dallas, TX 75235 **[105]**

Clement Ip, Department of Breast Surgery, Roswell Park Memorial Institute, 666 Elm Street, Buffalo, NY 14263 **[31]**

David Kessel, Departments of Medicine and Pharmacology, Wayne State University School of Medicine, 540 E. Canfield Street, Detroit, MI 48201 **[21]**

G.S. Kishore, Department of Breast Surgery, Roswell Park Memorial Institute, Buffalo, NY 14263 **[31]**

William L. McGuire, Department of Medicine, University of Texas Health Science Center, 7703 Floyd Curl Drive, San Antonio, TX 78284 **[71]**

Muriel Morisset, Unité d'Endocrinologie Cellulaire et Moléculaire (U 148), INSERM, 60, rue de Navacelles- 34100 Montpellier, France **[125]**

The number in brackets is the opening page number of the contributor's article.

Beverly Myers, Department of Pathology, Mt. Zion Hospital, 1600 Divisadero, San Francisco, CA 94115 **[3]**

J.K. Patel, Department of Breast Surgery, Roswell Park Memorial Institute, Buffalo, NY 14263 **[31]**

Kelly Patrick, Department of Internal Medicine, The University of Texas Health Science Center, 5323 Harry Hines Blvd., Dallas, TX 75235 **[105]**

Michael K. Robinson, Department of Immunochemistry Research, Evanston Hospital, 2650 Ridge Avenue, Evanston, IL 60201 **[47]**

Henri Rochefort, Unité d'Endocrinologie Cellulaire et Moléculaire (U 148), INSERM, 60, rue de Navacelles - 34100 Montpellier, France **[125]**

Ernest H. Rosenbaum, Department of Hematology-Oncology, Mt. Zion Hospital, 1600 Divisadero, San Francisco, CA 94115 **[3]**

Matthew Sakada, Department of Pathology, French Hospital, 4131 Geary Blvd., San Francisco, CA **[3]**

Edward F. Scanlon, Department of Surgery, Evanston Hospital, 2650 Ridge Avenue, Evanston, IL 60201 **[47]**

Georg F. Springer, Department of Immunochemistry Research, Evanston Hospital, 2650 Ridge Avenue, Evanston, IL 60201 **[47]**

Herta Tegtmeyer, Department of Immunochemistry Research, Evanston Hospital, 2650 Ridge Avenue, Evanston, IL 60201 **[47]**

Isabelle Touïtou, Unité d'Endocrinologie Cellulaire et Moléculaire (U 148), INSERM, 60, rue de Navacelles - 34100 Montpellier, France **[125]**

Tracy T. Trujillo, John Muir Cancer and Aging Research Institute, 2055 North Broadway, Walnut Creek, CA 94561 **[3]**

F. Vignon, Unité d' Endocrinologie Cellulaire et Moléculaire (U 148), INSERM, 60, rue de Navacelles - 34100 Montpellier, France **[125]**

David T. Zava, John Muir Aging and Cancer Institute, 2055 North Broadway, Walnut Creek, CA 94596 **[71]**

Preface

The Breast Cancer Working Group of the Organ Systems Program, National Cancer Institute, sponsored a Workshop through the Organ Systems Coordinating Center, entitled "Tumor Markers and Their Significance in the Management of Breast Cancer." The Workshop was held at the National Institutes of Health, Bethesda, Maryland. The Program Committee consisted of Angela Brodie and Thomas Dao (Co-Chairpersons), and Roberto Ceriani, Irma Russo, and Albert Segaloff. The Workshop program is reproduced as follows:

Session I   Circulating tumor markers

Role of circulating human mammary epithelial antigens as serum markers for breast cancer
Roberto Ceriani, M.D., Ph.D., John Muir Cancer & Aging Institute

Monoclonal antibodies, tests and breast cancer
William Feller, M.D., Ph.D., Georgetown University Hospital

Glycosyltransferases as tumor markers
David Kessel, Ph.D., Wayne State University

Sialyltransferase in serum and tumor tissue in women with breast cancer
Thomas Dao, M.D., Roswell Park Memorial Institute

Session II   Breast cancer antigens

Monoclonal antibodies, oncogenes, and human carcinomas
Jeffrey Schlom, Ph.D., National Cancer Institute

Monoclonal antibodies to surface antigens of the T47D human breast carcinoma cell line
Ricardo Mesa-Tejada, M.D., Columbia-Presbyterian Medical Center

Studies with a monoclonal antibody which defines a
tumor-associated antigen in human breast cancer
> Dean Edwards, Ph.D., University of Colorado

Serological analysis of human breast cancer with
human and mouse monoclonal antibodies
> Richard Cote, M.D., Memorial Sloan-Kettering
> Cancer Center

Session III   Estrogen metabolites and estrogen-induced proteins

Biochemical epidemiology of breast cancer
> Jack Fishman, Ph.D., Rockfeller University

Estrogen regulation of H59 in breast cancer *in vivo*
and *in vitro*
> Fred Hendler, M.D., Ph.D., University of
> Texas, Dallas

Estrogen-regulated proteins secreted by breast cancer cells
> Henri Rochefort, M.D., Ph.D., Montpellier,
> France

This volume contains a partial collection of manuscripts submitted by the participants. Four of them chose not to publish. A manuscript is included from Dr. Georg Springer, who was invited to give a talk at the Breast Cancer Working Group meeting on March 7th.

This book is dedicated to Dr. Albert Segaloff, who passed away on February 27, 1985, at the age of 68, at his home in New Orleans, Louisiana. Dr. Segaloff played a prominent role in the development of the National Cancer Institute's breast cancer programs, serving as chairman of the Cooperative Breast Cancer Group from 1956 to 1968, as a member of the Breast Cancer Task Force from 1966–1970, and as a member of the Breast Cancer Working Group until his death.

> Clement Ip, Ph.D.
> Scientific Administrator
> Breast Cancer Program
> Organ Systems Coordinating Center

I. Circulating Tumor Markers

Tumor Markers and Their Significance in the Management of Breast Cancer, pages 3–19
© **1986 Alan R. Liss, Inc.**

ROLE OF CIRCULATING HUMAN MAMMARY EPITHELIAL ANTIGENS (HME-Ags) AS SERUM MARKERS FOR BREAST CANCER*,**

Roberto L. Ceriani, M.D., Ph.D. ***, Ernest H. Rosenbaum, M.D.[2], Mark Chandler, B.A.[1] and Tracy T. Trujillo, B.S.[1], Beverly Myers, M.D.[2], Matthew Sakada, M.D.[3]
John Muir Cancer and Aging Research Inst., 2055 N. Broadway, Walnut Creek, CA 94561[1], Mt. Zion Hosp. San Francisco, CA[2], French Hosp., San Francisco, CA[3]

INTRODUCTION:

The idea of screening and following patients with breast cancer by a serum test is appealing from several points of view including its easiness, its economic advantages, its possibility of repeated sampling and its non-invasiveness. So strong and pervasive are these and other reasons that this approach has been continuously proposed, and perhaps with limited success, newer tests have been made available intermittently. As expected the aim to be achieved by every novel test, thus guaranteeing advantage over previous ones, has been greater specificity and higher sensitivity. In spite of the two latter proclaimed goals, by force or necessity, most tests available had to rely on less than ideal specificity (they are usually pan-carcinoma-detecting tests). In addition their sensitivity usually was restricted to a certain

ABBREVIATIONS: anti-HME = anti-human mammary epithelial antigen; CEA = carcinoembryonic antigen; HME-Ags = human mammary epithelial antigen; HMFG = human milk fat globule; LDH = lactic dehydrogenase; ng/ml = nanograms/ml; NPGP = non-penetrating glycoprotein.

** This work was supported by grants from the Dept. of Human Health Services, NIH, NCI, CA-39932 and 39933.

*** From whom reprints should be requested.

percentage of positivity in known breast cancer patients, even among those with important tumor load, thus yielding many false negatives.

In search for specificity the notion that breast tissue had differentiation antigens of its own (Ceriani et al., 1977) created newer expectations. These differentiation antigens, that we discovered and called human mammary epithelial antigens (HME-Ags), identified cell surface components of human breast epithelial cells that were found in every human breast cell line (Peterson et al., 1978) and human breast tumors (Sebesteny, et al., 1979; Peterson et al., 1981) tested to date. These components have been identified by rabbit antisera (anti-HME) created by injections of human milk fat globule membrane (HMFG) which are subsequently absorbed with human epithelial cells (Ceriani et al., 1977). In every instance rabbit antisera with surprisingly similar specificity were prepared that recognized 3 components of the breast epithelial cell membrane (Ceriani et al., 1977; Sasaki et al., 1981; Sasaki, Wara et al., 1981). These components were glycoproteins of apparent molecular weight of 150,000, 70,000 and 40,000 daltons (Ceriani et al., 1977; Sasaki et al., 1981). Anti-HME was used immediately to quantitate the presence of their corresponding antigens in a first generation radioimmunoassay (RIA) to measure HME-Ags on human breast epithelial cells (Sasaki et al., 1981). This RIA used a precipitation with protein-A-laden bacteria of immune complexes formed between anti-HME and its antigens. With this same assay it was possible to find high values of circulating HME-Ags in nude mice implanted with human breast carcinomas (Sasaki, Wara et al., 1981). Mice grafted with human non-breast tumors did not have HME-Ags in their sera (Sasaki, Wara et al., 1981). The fact that promoted HME-Ags as a serum-marker for breast cancer was that surgical removal of these human breast tumors in the nude mice eliminated the high titers of HME-Ags (Sasaki, Wara et al., 1981).

The potential value of these differentiation antigens of the breast prompted the search for a more sensitive RIA to measure the much lower serum levels to be expected in breast cancer patients. For this purpose a solid phase RIA was developed that used anti-HME

covalently bound to Sepharose-beads which bind HME-Ags
present in the breast cancer patient's serum (Ceriani et
al., 1982). These HME-Ags bound to the solid phase were
then measured by the radioiodine labelled polyclonal anti-
HME. A further refinement was the use of biotinilated
anti-HME that was in turn recognized by radioiodinated
avidin. With this assay it was possible to detect HME-Ags
levels in 75% of stage IV patients and in 25% of stages I
and II. Sera from non-breast cancer patients as well as
patients with benign breast lesions and normal women were
negative. In an effort to confirm the results obtained by
the RIA a very sensitive analytical technique was
developed to identify the breast HME-Ags that could be
present in the human serum (Ceriani et al., 1982). This
approach consisted of scavenging from the sera HME-Ags
with anti-HME bound to Sepharose-beads. The antigens on
the beads were then labelled in situ with radioiodine and
ultimately released with low pH. Thus very small amounts
of HME-Ags could be extracted from the serum, labelled and
then analyzed for molecular characteristics. By this
methodology, the 3 HME-Ags identified by anti-HME were
consistently recovered from breast cancer patient serum,
thus proving that these antigens are undoubtedly in
circulation. Applying a similar technique it was also
possible to recover from sera of breast cancer patients
the corresponding antigen of an anti-breast monoclonal
antibody that we recently prepared (Ceriani et al., 1983).
This monoclonal antibody was prepared by hybridization of
spleen cells of mice immunized with HMFG and has an
apparent molecular weight of 45,000 daltons. Thus it was
envisaged that possibly most, if not all, components of
the cell surface of breast epithelial cells are voided
into the circulation. In fact, a large molecular weight
component of the HMFG that were originally described
(Ceriani et al., 1983) has also been found in the
circulation of breast cancer patients (unpublished
results). This component (40,000 daltons, approximately
molecular weight) was called by us non-penetrating
glycoprotein (NPGP) and was found in the sera of breast
cancer patients in fragments of reduced molecular weight
(unpublished results).

Confirmatory evidence for our findings has come from other laboratories (Papsidero et al., 1984; Hilkens, et al., 1985) which using monoclonal antibodies have also detected breast epithelial cell components in the circulation of breast cancer patients. These findings of cell components in circulation are not isolated since less specific components of the breast epithelial cell have been detected in sera of breeast cancer patients. Among them sialytransferase (Ip and Dao, 1978) is one that has shown clinical application.

In this paper we describe comparative assays for HME-Ags, CEA and NPGP in longitudinally sampled breast and non-breast cancer patients. Specificity, sensitivity and predictive values for these assays as well as for LDH and alkaline phosphatase in serum are determined and guidelines for their future clinical use are presented.

MATERIALS, METHODS AND RESULTS

An important feature of a polyclonal antibody RIA of the type used is that it gathers its strength from specificity of the antibody for breast epithelial cells. This specificity was obtained in these antibodies by the repeated absorptions of the 40% ammonium precipitate of the rabbit antiserum, with several cellular materials. As previously mentioned (Sasaki et al., 1981), after each absorption the antiserum was again back tested to the absorbing cells for demonstration of its lack of cross-reactivity and to mammary epithelial cells to demonstrate its remaining titer.

The antiserum has been demonstrated to bind three components of the milk fat globule membrane (Ceriani et al., 1977; Sasaki et al., 1981), by affinity chromatography and double immunoprecipitations. These three components are different from another heavy molecular weight (NPGP) antigen of the human milk fat globule already described by us (Ceriani et al., 1983) and others. This antigen is present not only in breast

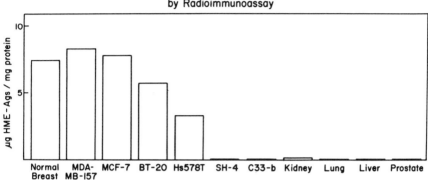

Fig. 1. Protein-A RIA for HME-Ags present in different human cell lines and tissues. MDA-MB-157, MCF-7, BT-20 and HS578T are human breast cancer cell lines, SH-4 a human melanoma cell line and C33-ba human cervical carcinoma cell line.

epithelial cells but in other secretory cells of the organism, thus it is absorbed by carcinoma cells used to absorb anti-HME.

To test for specificity of anti-HME, both a solid phase binding assay of the membranes of the cells used for absorption and a protein-A assay that we have already described (Sasaki et al., 1981) were used to obtain values for HME-Ags in several human tissues and cell lines. Figure 1 shows that HME-Ags were found in important quantities only in breast epithelial cells. Similar results were described previously by us (Sasaki et al., 1981).

In this study, to measure HME-Ags in breast cancer patient serum, a three-step competitive RIA was used which we have already described in detail (Ceriani et al., 1985). In brief, sera of normal controls, breast cancer

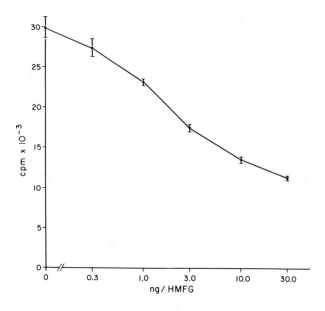

Fig. 2 Standard curve for dilutions of HMFG. Values are given for HMFG/protein equivalent in nanograms as detected by the RIA.

patients were drawn at Mt. Zion Hospital and frozen at -70 C until use. For the assay, immune complexes of HME-Ags and of the patients and control sera to the antisera were precipitated. The remaining anti-HME activity on the supernatant was then measured against HMFG bound onto a solid phase.

This RIA design was able to detect in a reproducible statistically significant fashion quantities of HME-Ags down to 1 ng/ml of HMFG equivalent protein. It should be taken into account that the cut off line for the present RIA is 100 ng/ml, and the dilution of the patients' sera used was 1 to 30. Therefore, if there was any values in the sera between 30 - 100 ng/ml, they would have been easily detected. The standard curves obtained were

reproducible in every assay; an example of one is
presented in figure 2. In some instances, values exceeded
the HME-Ags level interval detected by our standard
curves; these values were expressed as being above 300
nanograms per ml.

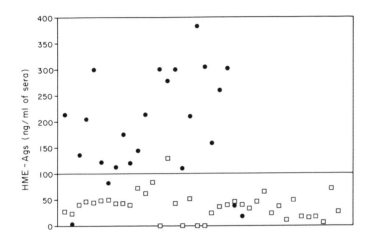

Fig. 3 HNE-Ags values for relapsing breast cancer
patients ● : and for relapsing non-breast cancer
patients □.

In a study for specificity, sera of 25 patients with
relapsing breast cancer were compared to the sera of 25
patients with relapsing non-breast cancer. As it can be
seen in figure 3, with only one exception, all the sera of
the non-breast cancer patients were below the 100
nanograms per ml cut off line for this assay. The only
exception found to date has been in a patient with lung
cancer whose value was 136 nanograms per ml. Thus, these
figures indicated the specificity of this test for breast
cancer patients as well as its low rate of false
negatives.

We had previously shown, using the different RIA
methodology and also through direct extraction of the

antigens from the serum and in situ labelling, that normal patients do not have HME-Ags antigens in circulation (Ceriani et al., 1982). Thus when assayed by our RIA, it can be shown that normal female sera give values well below 100 nanograms of HME-Ags per ml. which was considered background noise for this test and not real HME-Ags values. The average obtained for our controls was 22.4 ng/ml. In Table 1, these values are shown together with the values for the breast cancer patients studied to date and non-breast cancer patients. The latter are

Table 1

HME-Ags LEVEL IN BREAST TUMORS
NON-BREAST TUMORS AND CONTROLS

BREAST TUMORS (25)	202.6 ± 23.5
NORMAL CONTROLS (25)	22.7 ± 2.1
NON-BREAST TUMORS (38)	42.6 ± 3.9
Colon Ca (7)*	43.39**
Lymphoma (6)	46.00
Myeloma (2)	60.8
Ovary (8)	39.5
Melanoma (4)	22.6
Leukemia (2)	23.7
Pancreas (1)	39.9
Lung (3)	83.5
Larynx (1)	49.2
Endometrium (2)	27.8

* Number of cases in parentheses
** Plus or minus standard error of mean

separated into the different cancer types. It can be clearly seen that none of the averages for the non-breast cancer patients exceeds the cut-off line. In addition, in 25 cases with confirmed breast cancer in relapse, the serum levels of HME-Ags, lactose dehydrogenase (LDH) and alkaline phosphatase were compared (fig. 4). Since these patients are confirmed breast cancer patients, any values to the left of the central divider (which indicates the boundary between normalcy and disease value) will be those called false negative. It can be clearly seen that the HME-Ags is a test that results in a lower number of false negatives, and thus has a higher degree of specificity. This latter parameter as well as sensitivity and

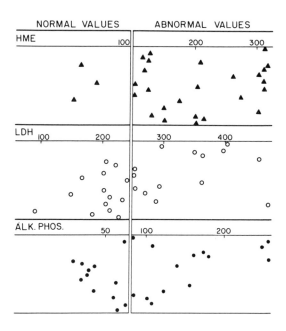

Fig. 4   Values for HME-Ags (HME), lactic dehydrogenase (LDH), and alkaline phosphatase (ALK. PHOS.) in 25 relapsing breast cancer patients.   The center line separates false negatives from true positives.

predictive value have been analyzed for all three blood
tests in the same samples and the results are depicted in
table 2. Sensitivity, specificity and predictive value
were substanially higher for the present RIA for the HME-
Ags test presented here than for alkaline phosphatase and
LDH.

Table 2
HME-Ags

SENSITIVITY	94%
SPECIFICITY	96%
PREDICTIVE VALUE FOR POSITIVE RESULTS	96%

LDH

SENSITIVITY	50%
SPECIFICITY	82%
PREDICTIVE VALUE FOR POSITIVE RESULTS	55%

ALKALINE PHOSPHATASE

SENSITIVITY	57%
SPECIFICITY	76%
PREDICTIVE VALUE FOR POSITIVE RESULTS	28%

The appreciable sensitivity obtained with the
present RIA allowed for the follow-up of breast cancer
patients in relapse. A series of breast cancer patients
in this condition were followed up with samples drawn
every one, two or three months while their clinical
condition was also recorded. Simultaneously, values for
CEA (Abbott CEA assay) were also obtained, the results are
demonstrated in fig. 5 and 6, which show the longitudinal
studies of HME-Ags. An increase in HME-Ags correlates

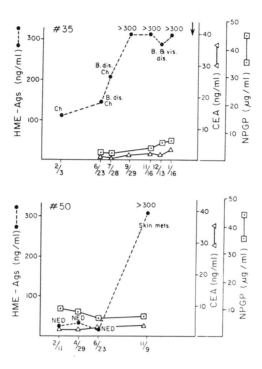

Fig. 5. Longitudinal serum levels in time of
HEM-Ags, CEA and NPGP in breast cancer patients.

with appearance of clinically certified relapse. In many
cases, HME-Ags were present while CEA was undetected. Two
types of correlations were found: i) HEM-Ags are elevated
during a period of relapsing metastases, while CEA is not
(fig. 5); and ii) HME-Ags detected during relapse
together with CEA, in patient #4, (fig. 6); and with a
lesser quantitative response, HME-Ags detected during
relapse much prior to CEA, in patient #11, (fig. 6). As a
corollary, it must be noticed that the HME-Ags values were
usually much larger than CEA in the cases where the latter
was present, and in some cases, HME-Ags preceded CEA in
appearance by several months.

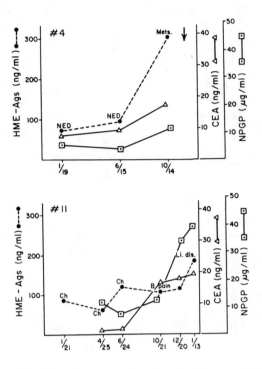

Fig. 6. Longitudinal serum levels in time of HME-Ags, CEA and NPGP in breast cancer patients.

We have previously reported on a monoclonal antibody capable of detecting a heavy molecular weight component present on human milk fat globule (NPGP) (Ceriani et al., 1983). Using these monoclonal antibodies, a radioimmunoassay was developed which was published in detail elsewhere (Ceriani et al., 1985). The sera of breast and non-breast cancer patients already tested for HME-Ags and CEA were also tested for NPGP. Many breast cancer patients although positive for HME-Ags, were negative for NPGP. In general, this latter assay had a lower sensitivity than the polyclonal assay for HME-Ags. When patients #35 and #50 (fig. 5), and patient #4 (fig. 6) were also studied for levels of NPGP in sequential sampling, the lack of sensitivity of the monoclonal assay was easy to observe. One of the patients with metastatic breast cancer had a distinctive increase in the levels of NPGP, with the appearance of bone pain, (see patient #11, fig. 6). Abnormal values of CEA and HME-Ags were also identified, approximately 4 months before the increase in NPGP.

DISCUSSION

The present RIA, although it detects HME-Ags similar to those we already published (Sasaki et al., 1981; Ceriani et al., 1982), uses a different approach. The former assay was a sandwich RIA that had as its drawbacks its non-competitive nature, the high radioactivity background given by the solid matrix used, and the large expense represented by the required quantitites of absorbed anti-serum to bind to the Sepharose beads. In the present RIA an antibody utilization approach is taken and the quantity of anti-serum to be used has been largely decreased. Further the present technology permits the deployment of all the RIA in micro titer plates.

The range of the assay down to 1 ng/ml compares favorably to most assays currently used in the clinical laboratory. Values somewhat larger than those obtained with the previous radioimmunoassay could be attributed either to a lesser antigen-antibody reaction as represented by the solid phase-liquid interaction of the former assay or by the more convenient use of micro-titer plates and non-specific absorptions of proteins.

We have established both in an experimental model and in the human the presence of HME-Ags in the circulation in breast cancer (Ceriani et al., 1982). We have given definite proof of their existence in the circulation by extraction methods (Ceriani et al., 1982) and their high levels in breast cancer patients by RIA. Their absence in non-breast cancer patients as demonstrated by very sensitive procedures has been also established (Ceriani et al., 1982). Again, this time they are shown to be present in the sera of breast cancer patients tested with an alternative methodology than the one used before. These results extend our previous findings and the larger series of patients in this study confirms without doubt that HME-Ags are present in high values in breast cancer patients. It is worth noting that in the meantime, with the use of monoclonal anibodies

against NPGP, other authors (Hilkens et al., 1985) have
found its antigens in circulation in breast cancer
patients. These assays, although imperfect, also confirm
our previous results. It is unfortunate that this
monoclonal antibody in fact detects an antigen with less
specificity than HME-Ags, such that it was only with the
use of HME-Ags that it was possible to clearly separate
the breast cancer patients from the non-breast cancer
patients, both in our previous study and now clearly in
our present one.

In regards to the specificity of this assay it can
be said that the use of a polyclonal antibody is
beneficial since any cross activity found can be easily
absorbed, while anti-HME titers still remain high to
permit the performance of the assay. In the case of
monoclonal antibodies, this is not a possibility.
The specificity for breast of anti-HME, with only one
exception has been very clearly demonstrated in this
paper. Further, compared to other proposed breast cancer
markers such as CEA, LDH or alkaline phosphatase, the
present assay was found to be far superior.

The value of the described assay in its present form
is clearly defined as a diagnostic and follow-up tool in
breast cancer. We have previously demonstrated the
presence of different cell surface components of the
normal breast epithelial cell in the circulation of breast
cancer patients (Ceiani et al., 1982). This paper extends
this concept further, and thus provides grounds to believe
that most if not all of the components of the cell
membrane of breast epithelial cells will be found
circulating in breast cancer patients, either intact or
denatured. In this regard, we have also found one cell
surface component of breast epithelial cells in the
circulation of breast cancer patients that is identified
by a monoclonal antibody; this component was present with
identical molecular weight to its native protein (Ceriani
et al., 1982). The three components identified by the
antisera used in the present assay also had conserved
their molecular weight; in contrast the antigen
corresponding to the monoclonal antibody to NPGP seems to
be denatured (unpublished results).

The possible denaturation of NPGP mentioned above could then be responsible for the irregular and insensitive results found for this antigen in the sera of breast cancer patients. Perhaps in different patients, due to local tumor conditions (necrosis, rapid growth, etc.) or circulatory conditions (hydrolyzing enzymes, kidney filtration, fast or slow clearance, etc.) levels of NPGP could become less reliable. Presently this matter is under investigation in our laboratory.

With procedures such as those described in this paper and in a previous one (Ceriani et al., 1982), it will be possible in the near future to identify and quantitate which components of the breast cancer epithelial cells are in circulation in the breast cancer patient. This approach will be very valuable for being able, by simple and non-invasive methods, to determine the antigenic composition of the cell surface of the breast tumor. If the oncologist wants to have the breast cancer patient imaged with labeled monoclonal antibodies or even later treated with any of the modalities introduced by monoclonal antibodies, an understanding of the antigenic composition of the cell surface of the tumor to be imaged or treated will thus be crucial. With our demonstration of the presence of such components in circulation and with the methodology developed for their identification and quantitation, this cell surface mapping of breast cancer cells using serum samples is becoming a reality.

Undoubtedly, early detection of a relapse in a breast cancer patient is of great importance to the oncologist so that appropriate treatment could be instituted as soon as possible. The present RIA can achieve this and further could be useful in detecting the results of radio- or chemotherapy. It could even be argued that residual tumor masses after surgery could also be detected by the present methodology.

Further, as improvements in the methodology for the detection of HME-Ags in the circulation become a reality, the possibility of having a screening test for the female population for breast cancer would only depend on the sensitivity and specificity of the assay. However, it could be postulated that screening would be greatly benefited by a simpler and unexpensive test. Thus, to achieve the latter goals, the present assay will have to be increased in sensitivity and simultaneously made less time consuming.

REFERENCES

Ceriani RL, Thompson KE, Peterson JA and Abraham S (1977). Surface differentiation antigens of human mammary epithelial cells carried by the human milk fat globule. Proc. Nat. Acad. Sci. (U.S.) 74:582.

Ceriani RL, Sasaki M, Sussman H, Wara WE and Blank EW (1982). Circulating human mammary epithelial antigens (HME-Ags) in breast cancer. Proc. Nat. Acad. Sci., U.S. 79:5421.

Ceriani RL, Peterson JA, Lee JY, Moncada FR and Blank EW (1983). Preparation and characterization of monoclonal antibodies to normal human breast epithelial cells. Som. Cell Genet. 9:415.

Ceriani RL, Rosenbaum EH, Chandler M and T Trujillo (1985). Human mammary epithelial antigens (HME-Ags) and other cancer markers in the serum of breast cancer patients. Submitted for publication.

Hilkens J, Kroezen V, Buijs F, Hilgers J, van Vliet M, de Voogd W, Bonfer J and Bruning PF (1985). MAM-6, A carcinoma associated marker: Prelimina breast cancer patients. In: International workshop of monoclonal antibodies and breast cancer, R. Ceriani, ed., M. Nijhoff, Publ. New York, N.Y., in press.

Ip C and Dao T (1978). Alterations in serum glycosyltransferases and 5'-nucleotidase in breast cancer patients. Cancer Res. 38:723.

Papsidero LD, Nemoto T, Croghan GA and Chu TM (1984). Expression of ductal carcinoma antigen in breast cancer sera as defined using monoclonal antibody F36122. Cancer Res. 44:4653.

Peterson JA, Buehring G, Taylor-Papadimitriou J and Ceriani RL (1978). Expression of human mammary epithelial (HME) antigens in primary cultures of normal and abnormal breast tissue. Int. J. Cancer 22:655.

Peterson JA, Bartholomew JC, Stampfer M and
    Ceriani RL (1981). Analysis of expression of
    human mammary epithelial antigens in normal and
    malignant breast cells at the single cell level
    by flow cytofluorimetry. Exp. Cell Biol. 49:1.
Sasaki M, Peterson JA and Ceriani RL (1981).
    Quantitation of human mammary epithelial
    antigens in cells cultured from normal and
    cancerous breast tissues. In Vitro 17:150.
Sasaki M, Peterson JA, Wara W and Ceriani RL
    (1981). Human mammary epithelial antigens
    (HME-Ags) in the circulation of nude mice
    implanted with breast and non-breast tumors.
    Cancer 48(11):2214.
Sebesteny A, Taylor-Papadimitriou J, Ceriani
    RL, Millis R, Schmitt C and Trevan D (1979).
    Primary human breast carcinomas transplantable
    in the nude mouse. J. Nat. Cancer Inst.
    63:1331.

Tumor Markers and Their Significance in the Management of Breast Cancer, pages 21–30
© **1986 Alan R. Liss, Inc.**

GLYCOSYLTRANSFERASES AS MARKER ENZYMES IN NEOPLASIA

David Kessel

Departments of Medicine and Pharmacology
Wayne State University School of Medicine
Detroit MI 48201

The glycosyltransferases are a series of enzymes which catalyze transfer of sugars onto appropriate protein or glycoprotein acceptors (Schachter, 1984). The presence of these enzymes in circulating blood has been reported, as has elevated levels of activity of certain transferases associated with pathologic states. Among the latter are a variety of malignant diseases. Many investigators have attempted to show correlations between the levels of different plasma glycosyltransferases vs. tumor burden, tumor prognosis, responsiveness to chemotherapy, and related phenomena. In this paper, I will briefly review these reports, and summarize results obtained by us and others regarding the usefulness of plasma glycosyltransferases as indices of disease status in patients with malignant disease.

MATERIALS AND METHODS

Fetuin was obtained from Calbiochem Inc., Los Angeles CA and from Sigma Chemical Co., St. Louis, MO. Fetuin was desialated via treatment with dilute sulfuric acid (Spiro, 1964). This procedure creates a galactose-terminal acceptor for measurement of sialyltransferase (Kessel & Allen 1975, Bernacki & Kim,1977, Bosmann & Hall,1974, Ip & Dao,1977) and fucosyltransferase (Khilanani et al,1977) activities. The terminal galactose residue could then be removed by sequential treatment with periodate and borohydride (Spiro,1964), to form an acceptor with an terminal N-acetylglucosamine residue, suitable for measurement of galactosyltransferase (Capel et al.1979, Chatterjee et al 1978), along with the activity of a 'core' fucosyltransferase (Wilson et al,1976, Khilanani et al 1978). Ampholytes and Ultrodex were obtained from LKB Instruments Inc., Silver Spring, MD. AG-1-X8, a purified form of the anion-exchange resin Dowex 1, was obtained from Biorad Laboratories, Richmond, CA.

UDP-[^{14}C] galactose (280 mCi/mmole), CMP-[^{14}C] sialic acid (9,217 and 18,900 mCi/mmole) and GDP-L-[^{14}C]fucose (174 Ci/mmole) were purchased from New England Nuclear Corp., Boston MA.

Plasma samples were obtained from normal donors, patients with granulocytic leukemias, breast cancer or other malignancies. Blood samples were chilled to 4° after collection in EDTA. Erythrocytes and platelets were removed by sequential centrifugations at 1500 x g for 10 min and for 10,000 x g for 20 min. The resulting plasmas were stored at -70° until used (< 10 days).

Total sialyltransferase activity was measured with a desialated fetuin acceptor, using CMP-sialic acid as substrate (Kessel & Allen,1975; Henderson & Kessel, 1977). Incorporation of label into the desialated fetuin acceptor was measured by elution of the reaction mixture through 0.5 x 1 cm columns of Dowex 1 (OH form). Free sialic acid and CMP-sialic acid are retained on the column, while the sialylated acceptor appears in the eluate.

Galactosyltransferase was measured using UDP-[^{14}C] Galactose as sugar donor, and asialo-agalactofetuin as acceptor (Chatterjee et al 1978), with one modification. After incubations, 200 μl assay mixtures were brought to 0.2 M with cysteine and eluted through 1 x 0.3 cm columns of Dowex AG1-X8 (OH form), which were then washed with 1 ml of water. Radioactivity in the eluate + washing was measured; this represents incorporation of label into the high mol. wt. acceptor. The cysteine serves to prevent formation of manganese dioxide dioxide which will interfere with column selectivity.

Fucosyltransferase activities were measured with two different acceptors: asialofetuin and asialo-agalactofetuin. The former acceptor has a -GlcNAc-Gal terminal sequence and can act as substrate for three plasma enzymes: the 2'-fucosyltransferase specified by the H gene (Chester et al;, 1976), a 3'-fucosyltransferase which transfers fucose onto

the 3^1 position of a GlcNAc residue subterminal to Gal
(Schenkel-Brunner et al, 1972); and a third enzyme which
forms an unknown linkage (Kessel et al, 1980). All of these
activities are inhibited by the SH reagent N-ethylmaleimide
(Chou et al, 1977). Asialo-agalactofetuin has a GlcNAc
terminal residue and acts as acceptor for a fourth fucosyltransferase (Wilson et al, 1976) which catalyzes formation of
a linkage between fucose and an internal GlcNAc residue.
This plasma enzyme activity is insensitive to N-
ethylmaleimide.

Total plasma fucosyltransferase activity was determined in
a mixture containing labeled GDP-fucose, an asialo-fetuin
acceptor.

Electrofocusing studies on plasma glycosyltransferases
were carried out using two procedures. A large-scale
separation was carried out using 2 ml plasma samples which
were focused for 16 hr on a 10 x 50 cm flat-bed of ultrafine
Sephadex over a pH range of 4-8. The gel bed was then
divided into 30 equal fractions and each eluted with 3 ml of
cold 20 mM HEPES buffer, pH 7.0. The fractions were then
used for measurement of sialyltransferase (Kessel et al,
1981) or fucosyltransferase (Kessel et al, 1980) activities
For measurement of plasma galactosyltransferase, which is
present at substantially higher levels than are the other
transferases, we devised a more rapid separation technique.

Rubber inserts were used to divide the focusing tray into
a bed size of 2.2 x 10.8 cm. The supporting gel was composed of 400 mg of Ultrodex suspended in 8 ml water, 250 µl
Ampholyte 4-6, 200 µl Ampholyte 6-8 and 50 µl Ampholyte 7-9.
This mixture was poured onto the plate, and additional
Ultrodex (85 mg) was sprinkled on the top of the gel to absorb excess fluid. The gel was finally smooth with a
plastic ruler. The gel bed temperature was kept at 4°, and
was focused for 2 hr at a constant power of 0.6 watt. The
plasma sample (50 µl) was then allowed to soak into a 2.2
x 0.2 cm region at the center of the gel. Focusing was
continued for an additional 60 min, and the gel divided into
approx. 0.8 cm sections with a plastic spatula. The pH of
the individual sections was determined, and the enzyme eluted with water. Activity was measured essentially as described by Davey et al. (1983a, 1983b). We later found that this
procedure could be adapted to the measurement of plasma
sialyl- and fucosyltransferases if high specific-

activity nucleotide-sugars were employed.

RESULTS AND DISCUSSION

Sialyltransferase studies

Elevated levels of plasma sialyltransferase were generally associated with the presence of neoplastic disease (Warren et al,1974; Kessel & Allen,1975; Dao et al,1980; Griffiths et al,1982; Henderson & Kessel,1977; Ip & Dao,1978).
But elevated enzyme levels were also found in inflammatory
disease, e.g., rheumatoid arthritis (Kessel & Allen, 1975).
Kaplan et al,(1983) also reported that inflammation causes
an elevation of plasma sialyltransferase levels in animals.
Plasma sialyltransferase provided a measure of tumor progression in neoplastic disease (Henderson & Kessel, 1977),
and of disease prognosis (Stewart et al,1982, 1983). But
the wide variation in plasma enzyme levels among normal controls, together with the effect of inflammation on the
results, argued against the likelihood that a measurement of
total plasma sialyltransferase would be a sensitive tumor
marker.

Electrofocusing studies showed the presence of at least
four distinct plasma sialyltransferase activities (Kessel et
al 1981). Enzymes with pI = 5.1 and 5.5 were found in all
control and pathologic plasmas. A third enzyme, with pI =
7.5, was also found in plasma of patients with rheumatoid
arthritis and other inflammatory diseases. A fourth species
with pI = 4.7 was found in the plasma of 12 patients with
primary or recurrent breast cancer. The electrofocusing
studies suggest that a specific sialyltransferase in plasma
is associated with the presence of neoplastic breast disease.

Release of sialyltransferase into plasma has been associated with the presence of neoplasia in animal models (Bernacki & Kim,1977; Ip & Dao,1977) and may represent a process
associated with shedding of membrane fragments and enzymes
during tumor invasion and metastasis (Yogeeswaran & Salk,
1981). The association of glycosyltransferases with membrane loci is well known (Shur & Roth,1975). Use of an assay with specificity for distinct enzyme species may provide
a useful diagnostic and prognostic assay. In this regard,

it is important to note that several workers have described
procedures for purification of sialyltransferases, and for
examination of the structures which are synthesized by the
different mammalian enzymes (Miyagi & Tsuiki, 1982; Paulson
et al, 1982; Sadler et al, 1979a, 1979b; Weinstein et al,
1982). The methodology described may be useful for
analogous studies on enzymes associated with human neoplasia.

Galactosyltransferase studies

Release of this enzyme activity into plasma has also been
associated with the presence of metastatic mammary tumors in
animal models (Chatterjee & Kimm, 1977; Chatterjee, 1979).
Elevated levels of plasma galactosyltransferase were found
in patients with ovarian tumors (Chatterjee et al., 1978;
Gauduchon et al., 1983), and with breast cancer (Paone et al,
1981).

In our studies of this plasma enzyme activity, we found
no uniform elevation in neoplastic disease. Furthermore,
electrofocusing studies showed no additional isoenzymes
aside from the band at pI 4-5, which were also found in normal plasmas. Plasma galactosyltransferase activity was suggested as a marker for ovarian cancer (Chatterjee, 1979).
In a more detailed study, Davey et al, (1983a) reported the
presence of at least 12 plasma isoenzymes, of which some or
all were elevated in neoplasia (Davey et al., 1983b). But
no unique plasma galactosyltransferase isoenzymes were associated with the presence of malignant disease. In contrast,
reports of a cancer-associated galactosyltransferase isoenzyme have been published (Weiser et al., 1975), but not yet
confirmed elsewhere.

Fucosyltransferase studies

Fucosyltransferase was suggested as a tumor marker for
bronchial (Ronquist & Nou, 1983) and colon cancer (Bauer et
al., 1978); its usefulness in breast cancer was limited (Ip
& Dao, 1978). We found a series of fucosyltransferase enzymes which were specific markers for marrow status in myelogenous leukemias.

Electrofocusing studies indicated an isoelectric point of

5.1 for the H gene-specified 2'-fucosyltransferase of plasma, while the 3'-fucosyltransferase focused at pH 5.5. Levels of the latter activity were markedly elevated in chronic myelogenous leukemias, and even more markedly elevated in blastic crisis (Shah-Reddy et al., 1982) which can be predicted from a sudden elevation in this enzyme level. A third N-ethylmaleimide sensitive plasma fucosyltransferase focused at pH 4.7. The plasma level of this enzyme reflected the presence of blast cells in the marrow of patients with acute myelogenous leukemias (Kessel et al., 1979). The isoelectric point of the N-ethylmaleimide resistant fucosyltransferase was pH 8.3. This enzyme catalyzes internal linkages (Wilson et al., 1976) and its activity in plasma is elevated during regeneration of normal marrow cells after successful chemotherapy of myelogenous leukemias (Kessel et al., 1978; Khilanani et al., 1978). Kuhns et al.(1980) reported that the activity of the H-gene associated 2'-fucosyltransferase activity in plasma was reduced in plasma of leukemic patients.

CONCLUSIONS

The potential use of plasma glycosyltransferases as marker enzymes for tumor diagnosis or prognosis remains uncertain. The type of high-resolution electrofocusing studies described by(Davey et al., 1983a) will be necessary to determine whether specific enzyme species are associated with neoplasia. If so, the development of more specific assay systems could result in a test procedure of clinical importance. At present, the relationship between plasma fucosyltransferases and marrow status in the leukemias looks promising. But the problems related to plasma enzyme purification and delineation of an appropriate clinical test procedure are substantial. The report of elevated levels of a specific plasma isoenzyme associated with breast cancer may prove helpful, if appropriate procedures can be devised for a more detailed identification of this enzyme activity.

REFERENCES

CH Bauer, WG Reutter, KP Erhart, E Kottgen and W Gerok. Decrease of human serum fucosyltransferase as an indicator of successful tumor therapy. Science 201: 1232-1222 (1978).

RJ Bernacki and U Kim. Concomitant elevations in serum sialyltransferase activity and sialic acid content in rats with metastasizing mammary tumors. Science 195:577-580, 1976.

HB Bosmann and TC Hall. Enzyme activity in invasive tumors of human breast and colon. Proc Nat Acad Sci 71:1833-1837, 1974.

ID Capel, M Jenner, MH Pinnock, HM Dorrell, DC Payne and DC Williams. Correlation between tumor size, metastatic spread, and galactosyl transferase activity in cyclophosphamide-treated mice bearing the Lewis Lung carcinoma. Oncology 36:242-244, 1979.

SK Chatterjee. Glycosyltransferases in metastasizing and non-metastasizing rat mammary tumors and release of these enzymes in the host sera. Europ J Cancer 15:1351-1356, 1979.

SK Chatterjee, M Bhattacharya and JJ Barlow. Correlation of UDP-galactose glycoprotein:galactosyltransferase levels in the sera with the clinical status of ovarian cancer patients. Cancer Lett 5:239-244, 1978.

SK Chatterjee and U Kim. Galactosyltransferase activity in metastasizing and non-metastasizing rat mammary carcinomas and its possible relationship with tumor cell surface antigen shedding. J Natl Cancer Inst 58:273-280, 1977.

MA Chester, AD Yates and WM Watkins. Phenyl β-D-galactosylpyranoside as an acceptor substrate for the blood-group H gene-associated guanosine diphosphate L-fucose:β-D-galactosyl α-2-L-fucosyltransferase. Eur. J. Biochem. 69, 583-592 (1976).

TH Chou, C Murphy and D Kessel. Selective inhibition of a plasma fucosyltransferase by N-ethylmaleimide. Biochem. Biophys. Res. Commun. 74, 1001-1007 (1977).

TL Dao, C Ip and J Patel. Serum sialyltransferase and 5'-nucleotidase as reliable biomarkers in women with breast cancer. J Nat Cancer Inst 65:529-534, 1980.

R Davey, R Bowen and J Cahill. The analysis of soluble galactosyltransferase isoenzyme patterns using high resolution agarose isoelectric focusing. Biochem. Internat. 6:643-651, 1983a.

RA Davey, RM Harvie, EJ Cahill and JA Levi. Serum galactosyltransferase isoenzymes as markers for solid tumors in humans. Eur. J. Cancer Clin. Oncol. 19:1043-1052, 1983b.

P Gauduchon, C Tillier, C Guyonnet, J-F Heron, E Bar-Guilloux and J-Y Le Thaler. Clinical value of serum glycoprotein galactosyltransferase levels in different histological types of ovarian cancer. Cancer Res 43:4491-4496, 1983.

J Griffiths and S Reynolds. Plasma sialyl transferase total and isoenzyme activity in the diagnosis of cancer of the colon. Clin Biochem 15:46-48, 1982.

M Henderson & D Kessel. Alterations in plasma sialyltransferase in patients with neoplastic disease. Cancer 39:1129-1134, 1977.

C Ip and T Dao. Increase in serum and tissue glycosyltransferases and glycosidases in tumor-bearing rats. Cancer Res 37: 3442-3447,1977.

C Ip and T Dao. Alterations in serum glycosyltransferases and 5'-nucleotidases in breast cancer patients. Cancer Res 38:723-728, 1978.

HA Kaplan, B Woloski, M Hellmann and JC Jamison. Studies on the effect of inflammation on rat liver and serum sialyltransferase. J Biol. Chem. 258:11505-11509, 1983.

D Kessel and J Allen. Elevated plasma sialyltransferase in the cancer patient. Cancer Res 35:670-672, 1975.

D Kessel, TH Chou & RC Coombes. Studies on sialyltransferase activities in plasma of patients with breast cancer. Eur J Cancer 17:1035-1040, 1981.

D Kessel, TH Chou, I Shah-Reddy, P Khilanani & I Mirchandani. Electrofocusing patterns of plasma fucosyltransferases in chronic granulocytic leukemia. Cancer Res 40:3576-3578, 1980.

D Kessel, P Khilanani & TH Chou. Levels of two plasma fucosyltransferases as an index of disease status in acute myelogenous leukemias. Cancer Treatment Repts 62:147-149, 1978.

D Kessel, V Ratanatharathorn & TH Chou. Electrofocusing patterns of fucosyltransferases in plasma of patients with neoplastic disease. Cancer Res 39:3377-3380, 1979.

P Khilanani, TH Chou & D Kessel. Plasma guanosine diphosphate-L-fucose:N-acetylglucosaminide fucosyltransferase as an index of bone marrow hyperplasia after chemotherapy. Cancer Res. 38:181-184, 1978.

P Khilanani, TH Chou, PL Lomen & D Kessel. Variation of levels of plasma guanosine diphosphate L-fucose:β-D-galactosyl α-2-L-fucosyltransferase in acute adult leukemia. Cancer Res 37:2557-2559, 1977.

WJ Kuhns, RTD Oliver, WM Watkins and P Greenwell. Leukemia-induced alterations of serum glycosyltransferase enzymes. Cancer Res. 40: 268-275 (1980).

T Miyagi and S Tsuiki. Purification and characterization of β-galactoside (α2-6)sialyltransferase from rat liver and hepatoma. Eur. J. Biochem. 126:253-261, 1982.

JF Paone, RR Baker, TP Waalkes and JH Shaper. Sequential galactosyltransferase and CEA levels in advanced breast cancer. J Surg Res 31:269-273,1981.

JC Paulson, J Weinstein and U de Souza-e-Silva. Identification of a Gal β1-3GlcNac α2-3 sialyltransferase in rat liver. J. Biol. Chem. 257:4034-4037, 1982

G Ronquist and E Nou. Serum sialyltransferase and fucosyltransferase activities in patients with bronchial carcinoma. Cancer 52:1679-1683, 1983.

JE Sadler, JL Rearick and RL Hill. Purification to homogeneity and enzymatic characterization of an αN-acetylgalactosaminide α2-6 sialyltransferase from porcine submaxillary glands. J. Biol. Chem. 254:5934-5941 (1979a).

JE Sadler, JL Rearick, JC Paulson and RL Hill. Purification to homogeneity of a β-galactoside α2-3-sialyltransferase and partial purification of an α-N-acetylgalactosaminide α2-6 sialyltransferase from porcine submaxillary glands. J. Biol. Chem. 254:4434-4443 (1979b).

H Schachter. Glycoproteins: their structure, biosynthesis and possible clinical implications. Clin Biochem 17:3-14, 1984.

I Shah-Reddy, D Kessel, TH Chou, I Mirchandani & U Khilanani. Plasma fucosyltransferase as an indicator of imminent blastic crisis. Am J Hematol 12:29-37, 1982.

H Schenkel-Brunner, MA Chester and WM Watkins. α-L-fucosyltransferases in human serum from donors of different ABO, secretor and Lewis blood-group phenotypes. Eur. J. Cancer 30, 267-277 (1972).

BD Shur and S Roth. Cell surface glycosyltransferases. Biochim Biophys Acta 415: 473-512, 1975.

RG Spiro. Periodate oxidation of the glycoprotein fetuin. J Biol Chem 239:567-573, 1964.

J Stewart, RB Rubens, S Hoare, RD Bulbrook & D Kessel. Serum sialyltransferase levels in patients with metastatic breast cancer treated by chemotherapy. Br J Cancer, 46:208-212, 1982.

J Stewart, R Rubens, R Millis, J Hayward, S Hoare, R Bulbrook & D Kessel. Post-operative serum sialyltransferase levels and prognosis in breast cancer. Breast Cancer Res and Treatment, 3:225-230, 1983.

L Warren, JP Fuhrer, CA Buck & EF Walborg, Jr. Membrane glycoproteins in normal and virus-transformed cells.

Miami Winter Symposia 8:1-21, 1974.

J Weinstein, U de Souza-e-Silva and JC Paulson. Purification of a Galβ1-4GlcNac α2-6 sialyltransferase and a galβ1-3(4)GlcNac α2-3 sialyltransferase to homogeneity from rat liver. J. Biol. Chem. 257:13835-13844 (1982).

MM Weiser, DK Podolsky and KJ Isselbacher. Cancer-associated isoenzyme of serum galactosyltransferase. Proc Nat Acad Sci 73:1319-1322, 1976.

G Yogeeswaran and PL Salk. Metastatic potential is positively correlated with cell surface sialylation of cultured murine tumor cell lines. Science 212:1514-1516, 1981.

JR Wilson, D Williams and H Schachter. The control of glycoprotein synthesis: N-acetylglucosamine linkage to a mannose residue as a signal for the attachment of L-fucose to the asparagine-linked N-acetylglucosamine residue of glycopeptide from α acid glycoprotein. Biochem. Biophys. Res. Commun. 72, 909-916 (1976).

Tumor Markers and Their Significance in the Management of Breast Cancer, pages 31–43

SERUM AND TUMOR SIALYLTRANSFERASE ACTIVITIES IN WOMEN WITH BREAST CANCER

T.L Dao, C. Ip, J.K. Patel, and G.S. Kishore

Department of Breast Surgery, Roswell Park Memorial Institute, Buffalo, N.Y. 14263

It is well-documented that neoplastic transformation of cells is accompanied by changes in the chemical composition of plasma membrane glycoconjugates. One aspect of such an alteration is an increase in the level of sialic acid on the cell surface (Warren, et al., 1972; Van Beek, et al., 1973). The presence of sialic acid in the cell surface glycoconjugates can influence a variety of biological properties, including electrokinetic potential of the cell (Forrester, et al., 1964), membrane permeability (Glick, and Githens, 1965), immunogenicity (Betesi, et al., 1971; Simmons, et al., 1971), as well as intercellular recognition and adhesion (Edelman, et al., 1976). Much significance has been attributed to the changes in the glycocalyx sialic acid for the abnormal behavior of cancer cells, as exemplified by invasiveness, metastasis and loss of contact inhibition of growth (Emmelot, 1973).

Sialyltransferase is the enzyme responsible for the transfer of the sugar from CMP-sialic acid to the appropriate substrate for the formation of a sialo-glycoconjugate. It is conceivable that elevated levels of cellular sialyltransferase could lead to an enhancement in the sialiation process. Changes in the total activities of various glycosyltransferases have been reported in human tumors, although the significance still remains unclear at the present time. Kessel and coworkers (1977) have demonstrated that increased levels of fucosyltransferases are associated with the primary tumor site (breast, ovary and colon), whereas sialyltransferase and galactosyltransferase activities are often higher at the tumor-host tissue interface. Chatterjee, et al. (1979) have shown that galactosyltransferase activity in ovarian tumors is higher than in normal ovaries. Likewise, sialyltransferase levels in breast and colon malignant tissues were also found by Bosmann and Hall (1974) to be higher than that in normal counterparts. The significance of the elevated sialyltransferase in the tumor tissue, however, is not yet understood.

Elevated serum sialyltransferase in women with primary or metastatic breast cancer has been demonstrated by several investigators (Kessel and Allen, 1975; Henderson, et al., 1977). In an earlier publication, we reported that serum levels of sialyltransferase and 5'-nucleotidase were reliable biomarkers in women with breast cancer. Our study demonstrated a significant correlation between the changes in the serum levels of these two enzymes and the course of the disease in women with metastatic breast cancer receiving treatment. Thus, the serum levels of these two enzymes rose or declined parallel to the progression or regression of the disease, respectively, in response to treatment. In women with primary operable stage I and II breast cancer, mastectomy caused a rapid fall of the elevated enzyme levels to within the normal range in all patients with stage I breast cancer, but not in those with stage II disease (Dao, et al., 1980).

The objective of the present study is to determine whether there is a correlation between tumor and serum sialyltransferase in women undergoing mastectomy for the treatment of primary breast cancer. We also wish to examine the presence or absence of a definite association between the content of the enzyme activities in the tumor and the extent of axillary **lymph node** metastases in these patients.

MATERIALS AND METHODS

Materials. CMP-[4,5,6,7,8,9-^{14}C]sialic acid (specific activity, 218 mCi/mole) was purchased from Amersham Corp., Arlington Height, IL. Fetuin was purchased from the Grand Island Biological Co., Grand Island, New York. Sialic acid-free fetuin was prepared by mild acid hydrolysis of fetuin, as described by Spiro (1960).

Tissue preparation. Human tumor specimens were acquired at surgery, trimmed of connective tissue and fat, and placed immediately in liquid nitrogen. They were stored at $-70°$ until ready for use. The frozen tissue was pulverized and homogenized in 5 volumes of ice-cold 0.14M KCl with a motor-driven Potter-Elvehjem homogenizer fitted with a Teflon pestle. The crude homogenate was filtered through cheesecloth. All subsequent differential centrifugation procedures were carried out at $4°$. Nuclei and cell debris were sedimented after low speed centrifugation at 1,000 x $\underline{g}$ for 10 minutes. Mitochondria were removed by centrifugation at 7,000 x $\underline{g}$ for 15 minutes. The supernatent was then spun at 105,000 x $\underline{g}$ for 60 minutes to separate the microsomal and cytosolic fractions. Routine sialyltransferase assays were determined with the microsomal pellet that was resuspended in 0.14M KCl to a protein concentration of 2-3 mg/ml. Protein was determined by the method of Lowry, et al. (1951).

Sialyltransferase assay. The incubation mixture contained 50 μl of tissue extract, 500 μg of sialic acid-free fetuin, 1 nmole CMP-[^{14}C]sialic acid (approximately 4.8×10^5 dpm), 1 mM $MnCl_2$, 1 mM uridine triphosphate (to inhibit CMP-sialic acid hydrolase), 0.1% Triton X-100, 20 mM Tris-maleate buffer (pH 7.0), in a final volume of 150 μl. To determine the endogenous activity, desialated fetuin was omitted in the mixture. Reaction was carried out at $37°$ for 60 minutes. Determination of the radioactivity incorporated into desialated fetuin has been described in detail previously by the authors (Ip, et al., 1978). Sialyltransferase activities are reported as calculated exogenous activities, i.e., total (in the presence of desialated fetuin) minus endogenous (in the absence of desialated fetuin) activities.

RESULTS

Sialyltransferase activities in breast tumors.
Figure 1 depicts the subcellular distribution of sialyltransferase in a representative human breast tumor. The width of the column along the abscissa indicates the percentage of protein recovered in each subcellular fraction, while the height of the column projects the relative specific activity of the enzyme with respect to the homo-

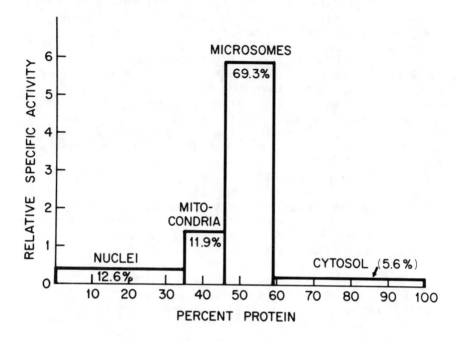

Fig. 1. Subcellular distribution of sialyltransferase in a representative human breast tumor.

genate. (The specific activity of sialyltransferase in the homogenate was set as 1.0.) Thus, the area enclosed by each column represents the total activity of sialyltransferase in each subcellular fraction. It can be seen that about 65-70% of the sialyltransferase was concentrated in the microsomes. In all subsequent routine assays, sialyltransferase was determined only in the microsomal pellet, so as to avoid excessive degradation of CMP-sialic acid by hydrolases, which normally would sediment with the nuclear and mitochrondrial fraction (results not shown).

The results of this study show a wide range of tumor sialyltransferase activities in the tumors. In order to rule out the possibility that low sialyltransferase activity in certain tumors was due to the presence of an inhibitor, we performed mixed-assay experiments involving tumor extracts with high and low enzyme levels in the same reaction tube. Results from these studies (table 1) demonstrated that sialyltransferase activities were additive in nature, suggesting that changes in enzyme levels probably reflected changes in the amount of enzyme protein. Measurement of CMP-sialic acid hydrolysis in the reaction mixture using tumor microsomal extract showed that <5% of substrate was degraded to sialic acid during incubation and that this activity was not related to the sialyltransferase levels (results not shown). It is therefore unlikely that the wide variation in sialyltransferase activities could be accounted for by degradation of the nucleotide-sugar donor.

TABLE 1. Assay of sialyltransferase activities in mixtures of microsomal extract from different breast tumors.

Experiments	Microsomal extract		Sialyltransferase activity	
	Tumor A*	Tumor B	Experimental	Theoretical
	(μl)		(pmoles/60 min)	
1	50	--	142	--
	--	50	18	--
	25	25	74	80
2	50	--	172	--
	--	50	48	--
	25	25	116	110
3	50	--	104	--
	--	50	12	--
	25	25	56	58

*Tumor A had higher sialyltransferase activity than tumor B. Each experiment consists of 2 different tumors, identified as tumor A and tumor B.

Sialyltransferase in serum and breast tumors. The tumor microsomal sialyltransferase activities in 35 primary breast cancer patients shows a wide range from 6-1238 pmol/mg protein/hr. The median enzyme activities in the tumors for this particular population was 90. Table 2 shows the tumor microsomal sialyltransferase activities as related to the number of axillary lymph node metastases found in 35 breast cancer patients at the time of mastectomy. In view of the wide range of enzyme activities observed, the patients were divided into 4 groups, according to the contents of their tumor sialyltransferase activities. The data show that tumors having sialyltransferase activities above the median of 90 appear to be associated with a higher number of nodal metastases in these patients. Of the 18 patients whose tumor sialyltransferase activities were below 90, 8 had no axillary nodal metastasis, 10 had metastasis in the lymph nodes, but only 1 had metastasis in more than 4 lymph nodes. In contrast, of the 17 patients whose tumor sialyltransferase activities were above the median of 90, 14 had positive lymph nodes (82.3%) and only 3 were negative for lymph node metastasis. Although the number of patients in this series is small, the data are strongly suggestive of a correlation between the level of tumor sialyltransferase activities and the invasiveness of the tumor.

TABLE 2. Relationship between tumor sialyltransferase activities and extent of lymph node metastasis.

SIALYLTRANSFERASE ACTIVITY*	NO. OF TUMORS	LYMPH NODE METASTASIS		
		0	1-3	>4
<50	11	5 (45%)	6 (55%)	0
51-90	7	3 (43%)	3 (43%)	1 (14%)
91-500	15	3 (20%)	4 (27%)	8 (53%)
>500	2	0	0	2 (100%)

*pmol/mg protein/hr

Table 3 discloses data on the levels of serum and tumor sialyltransferase activities in 35 patients with primary, potentially curable breast cancer. The sera from these patients was drawn 2-5 days prior to surgery. Tumors were obtained immediately after surgery, placed in liquid nitrogen, and processed for analysis of the microsomal enzyme, as described in "Methods and Materials". The results suggest that there is a correlation between the level of serum and breast tumor microsomal sialyltransferase activities in these patients. It appears that the increase in the serum enzyme levels is accompanied by a rise in tumor sialyltransferase activities. The number of patients in this study is too small to draw significant conclusions.

TABLE 3. Serum and tumor sialyltransferase in women with breast cancer.

| No. of Pts.* | Sialyltransferase Activities (pmol/mg protein/hr) | | | |
| | Serum | | Tumor | |
	Range	Mean	Range	Mean
5	6.0- 7.9	7.3	7.0- 250.0	72.0
8	8.0-10.9	9.7	6.0- 274.0	100.4
16	11.0-12.9	11.6	36.0-1238.0	275.3
6	13.0-18.9	15.9	54.0- 380.0	190.8

*Total number of patients: 35

Table 4 shows a comparison of tumor sialyltransferase activities in 35 patients with primary breast cancer with the levels found in 35 patients with metastatic cancer. It can be seen that there is an absence of tumors with low enzyme activities (<50) and increased activities in the metastatic tumors.

TABLE 4. Statistical distribution of sialyltransferase activities in human breast tumors.

| Tumor | Sialyltransferase Activity (pmoles/mg protein/hr) | | | | |
	<50	50-100	100-500	>500	TOTAL
Primary	11 (57%)	9 (26%)	13 (34.3%)	2 (5.7%)	35
Metastatic	--	15 (43%)	17 (48.6%)	3 (8.6%)	35

Serum sialyltransferase activities in patients with potentially curable breast cancer before and after surgery. To date, a total of 203 women with Stage I or II potentially curable breast cancer, of which 40 patients had wide local excision and axillary lymph node dissection (since 1981), and 163 had modified radical mastectomy, were followed in this study. Table 5 summarizes the data on the effect of the removal of the primary tumor on the levels of serum sialyltransferase in 162 patients with breast cancer.

TABLE 5. Serum sialyltransferase activities in women with breast cancer following mastectomy

Ax. lymph nodes	No. Pts.*	No. patients with normal sialyltransferase activities postoperatively	
		14 DAYS	>6 MONTHS
NEGATIVE	55 (20)	47 (85%)	47 (85%)
1-3	49† (14)	25 (51%)	42 (85%)
>4	58† (7)	15 (25%)	26 (45%)
TOTAL:	162 (41)		

*No. of patients with elevated sialyltransferase levels prior to surgery. Number in parentheses is the no. of patients with serum sialyltransferase levels within the normal range prior to surgery.

†Patients received adjuvant therapy, including either chemotherapy or endocrine ablations.

Serum sialyltransferase activities were measured before, 7-14 days after surgery, and regularly at 3-month intervals thereafter. The serum enzyme levels were elevated above the normal range in 55 patients with Stage I breast cancer (those without axillary lymph node metastasis) before mastectomy, and the levels declined to within the normal range in 47 patients (85%) within 14 days after surgical removal of the primary tumor. The levels remained within the normal range in these patients 6 months after surgery. In patients with 1-3 positive nodes, only 25 (51%) had the enzyme return to normal levels following surgery. However, at six months, 42 (85%) had levels within the normal range, following the administration of adjuvant therapy. In patients having >4 nodes positive, only 15 (25%) had normal levels two weeks following surgery and in only 26 (45%) were enzyme levels within the normal range at 6 months, despite the administration of adjuvant therapy. Of the 55 patients having negative nodes, in 8 patients, whose preoperative serum sialyltransferase levels were 15.8, 11.9, 13.8, 12.5, 14.1, 10.9, 12.4, and 11.0, enzyme levels failed to decline to normal levels, either immediately after surgery, at 6 months, or thereafter, and all these patients subsequently developed pulmonary metastasis, ranging from 10-18 months after mastectomy. The data shown in the following two tables illustrate this rather significant finding, which suggests that the enzyme levels may be a sensitive parameter for early and clinically undetected metastasis.

TABLE 6. Patient A.E. (55 years of age; mastectomy on 12/14/79; 0/31 lymph nodes positive).

	Sialyltransferase	5'-Nucleotidase
Preoperative	15.8	35.6
Postoperative		
10 days	13.9	33.1
3 months	13.5	27.0
6 months	13.5	28.0
9 months	13.2	24.3

Pulmonary metastasis detected 10 months after surgery.

TABLE 7. Patient D.H. (62 years of age; mastectomy on 7/3/79; 0/19 lymph nodes positive).

	Sialyltransferase	5'-Nucleotidase
Preoperative	11.9	34.6
Postoperative		
14 days	14.1	26.4
3 months	14.2	35.0
6 months	10.1	22.1
12 months	10.6	24.0
15 months	12.7	26.0
18 months	11.1	24.0
21 months	12.2	26.8

Chest X-ray at 15 months revealed the presence of bilateral pulmonary metastasis.

The remaining 47 patients continued to have "normal" serum sialyltransferase and they were disease-free between 7-84 months. The group of 20 patients in which preoperative enzyme levels were not elevated has been followed for a period of between 9 and 78 months following surgery. Only two patients showed a rise of the enzyme level above the normal range, one to 12.5 and the other to 11.5, at 36 and 40 months postoperatively, respectively. Both patients had clinical evidence of bone and lung metastasis at 38 and 43 months postoperatively. The follow-up of patients with axillary lymph node metastasis will be published in detail in a separate paper.

DISCUSSION

Our experiment demonstrated that breast tumor sialyltransferase is mostly concentrated in the microsomes. This is in agreement with previous studies in the liver which showed that intracellular glycosyltransferases are located primarily in the endoplasmic reticulum (Oliver, et al., 1975) and the Golgi complex (Schachter, et al., 1970). Recent biochemical and electron microscopic evidence, however, indicates that these enzymes are also present at the cell surface (Shur and Roth, 1975). It should be pointed out that we might also be measuring some "ecto-sialyltransferase" activity in our assays, since the microsomal preparation which we used as the enzyme source was contaminated by plasma membrane fragments.

The range as well as the statistical distribution of the enzyme activities appears to be similar in both the primary and metastatic tumors. Our results suggest that the changes in sialyltransferase activities in the tumors are probably due to alterations in the quantity of enzyme protein. Ingraham and Alhadeff (1978) suggested that inhibitor(s) of sialyltransferase might be present in cancerous liver tissues. The "inhibitor" could be in the form of increased levels of bound sialic acid in the tumor. We have found that the amount of bound sialic acid in the microsomal protein was not correlated (either directly or inversely) with the microsomal sialyltransferase activities (results not shown). It is therefore unlikely that the wide variation in sialyltransferase activities could be accounted for by the end product inhibition.

Preliminary analysis of data from the rather small series of patients suggests that tumors containing "high" levels of sialyltransferase activities appear to be more invasive, as indicated by the number of axillary lymph nodal metastases. The significance of this observation, however, must necessarily be confirmed by a much larger series, since no statistical analysis can be meaningfully made with the number of tumors in the present study. The measurement of serum sialyltransferase activities in this series of 35 patients with breast cancer suggests that there is a parallel between the levels of serum and tumor enzyme activities. Our data show that as the serum levels of sialyltransferase activities rose, there was a corresponding increase in the tumor enzyme activities. Again, this observation from a small series of patients must be substantiated by a study in a large number of patients.

Perhaps the most significant observation in this study is the finding that the level of sialyltransferase activity may indeed be a biochemical marker for the presence or absence of micrometastasis. The persistent elevation of the enzyme activities after mastectomy in eight patients without axillary lymph node metastasis that led to subsequent clinical evidence of the presence of visceral metastasis strongly indicates that the enzyme activities are in fact a sensitive parameter for detection of early and undetectable metastasis.

However, it should be noted that the reliability of a biochemical method can always be questioned, since the results may not be consistent, because of the multiplicity of sialyltransferases involved. Another difficulty is that interpretation of the enzymic data, especially on circulating sialyltransferase, may be affected by external parameters, such as medications and diet, which may possibly influence enzyme activity. Therefore, the development of a radioimmunoassay method is desirable, since it would provide consistently reliable and accurate measurements. In recent years, we have been working on the development of an RIA technique, based on monoclonal antibody technology. Purification of the enzyme has been completed and we are now developing monoclonal antibodies to sialyltransferase. We also wish to investigate whether this new ELISA method for measurement of the enzyme levels is specific to breast cancer or whether it is a general assay method that would be capable of detecting other types of cancer as well.

REFERENCES

Bekesi JG, St. Arneault G, Holland JF (1971). Increase of leukemia L1210 immunogenicity by Vibrio cholerae neuraminidase treatment. Cancer Res 31:2130-2132.

Bosmann HB, Hall TC (1974). Enzyme activity in invasive tumors of human breast and colon. Proc Natl Acad Sci USA 71:1833-1837.

Chatterjee SK, Bhattacharya M, Barlow JJ (1979). Glycosyltransferase and glycosidase activities in ovarian cancer patients. Cancer Res 39:1943-1951.

Dao TL, Ip C, Patel J (1980). Serum sialyltransferase and 5'-nucleotidase as reliable biomarkers in women with breast cancer. J Natl Cancer Inst 65:529-534.

Edelman GM (1976). Surface modulation in cell recognition and cell growth. Science 192:218-226.

Emmelot P (1973). Biochemical properties of normal and neoplastic cell surface. A review. Eur J Cancer 9:319-333.

Forrester JA, Ambrose EJ, Stoker MGP (1964). Microelectrophoresis of normal and transformed clones of hamster kidney fibroblasts. Nature 201:945-946.

Glick JL, Githens S (1965). Role of sialic acid in potassium transport of L1210 leukaemia cells. Nature 208:88.

Henderson M, Kessel D (1977). Alterations in plasma sialyltransferse levels in patients with neoplastic disease. Cancer 39:1129-1134.

Ingraham HA, Alhadeff JA (1978). Characterization of sialyltransferase in noncancerous and neoplastic human liver tissue. J Natl Cancer Inst 61:1371-1374.

Ip C, Dao TL (1978). Alterations in serum glycosyltransferases and 5'-nucleotidase in breast cancer patients. Cancer Res 38:723-728.

Kessel D, Allen J (1975). Elevated plasma sialyltransferase in the cancer patient. Cancer Res 35:670-672.

Kessel D, Sykes E, Henderson M (1977). Glycosyltransferase levels in tumors metastatic to liver and in uninvolved liver tissue. J Natl Cancer Inst 59:29-32.

Lowry OH, Rosebrough NJ, Farr AL, Randall RJ (1951). Protein measurement with the folin phenol reagent. J Biol Chem 193:265-275.

Oliver GJA, Harrison J, Hemming FW (1975). The mannosylation of dolichol-diphosphate oligosaccharides in relation to the formation of oligosaccharides and

glycoproteins in pig-liver endoplasmic reticulum.
Eur J Biochem 58:223-229.

Schachter H, Jabbal I, Hudgin RL, Pinteric L, McGuire EJ,
Roseman S (1970). Intracellular localization of liver
sugar nucleotide glycoprotein glycosyltransferases in
a Golgi-rich fraction. J Biol Chem 245:1090-1100.

Shur BD, Roth S (1975). Cell surface glycosyltransferases.
Biochim Biophys Acta 415:473-512.

Simmons RL, Rios A, Ray PK, Lundgren G (1971). Effect of
neuraminidase on growth of a 3-methylcholanthrene-
induced fibrosarcoma in normal and immunosuppressed
syngeneic mice. J Natl Cancer Inst 47:1087-1094.

Spiro RG (1960). Studies on fetuin, a glycoprotein of
fetal serum. J Biol Chem 235:2860-2869.

Van Beek WP, Smets LA, Emmelot P (1973). Increased sialic
acid density in surface glycoprotein of transformed and
malignant cells - a general phenomenon? Cancer Res
33:2913-2922.

Warren L, Fuhrer JP, Buck CA (1972). Surface glycoproteins
of normal and transformed cells: a difference determined
by sialic acid and a growth-dependent sialyltransferase.
Proc Natl Acad Sci USA 69:1838-1842.

II. Breast Cancer Antigens

**Tumor Markers and Their Significance in the Management
of Breast Cancer, pages 47–70**
© 1986 Alan R. Liss, Inc.

THE FUNDAMENTAL AND DIAGNOSTIC ROLE OF T AND Tn ANTIGENS IN
BREAST CARCINOMA AT THE EARLIEST HISTOLOGIC STAGE AND
THROUGHOUT

Georg F. Springer, Parimal R. Desai, Michael K.
Robinson, Herta Tegtmeyer and Edward F. Scanlon

Immunochemistry Research (G.F.S., P.R.D., M.K.R.,
H.T.), Evanston Hosp., Northwestern University,
Depts. of Surgery (G.F.S, P.R.D., M.K.R., E.F.S.)
and Microbiology-Immunology (G.F.S.), Evanston,
IL   60201

INTRODUCTION

A decade ago, we identified two carcinoma (CA)-associ-
ated antigens, T(Thomsen-Friedenreich) and Tn,that apparently
do not occur in immunoreactive form in healthy or in non-CA
diseased adult human tissues (Springer et al., 1974, 1975).
Until then, T and Tn had been studied only in relation to
blood groups and no connection with CA was suspected. All
humans have antibodies to both T and Tn antigens (Friedenreich, 1930; Burnet and Anderson, 1947; Dausset et al., 1959);
hence, T and Tn are thought not to be oncofetal antigens.
However, we recently found T- and Tn-specific structures to
occur transiently during early fetal development (Springer
et al., 1984; Klein-Szanto, A. and Springer, G.F., to be published).

Tn is the immediate precursor of T in its biosynthesis;
epitopes of both are, in turn, immediate precursors of the
MN blood group antigens (Springer and Desai, 1974, 1975;
Springer et al., 1976b; Cartron et al., 1978; Desai and
Springer, 1979, 1980) and distant precursors in other complex
O-glycosidically linked carbohydrate chains (Lloyd and Kabat,
1968). Both the T and Tn epitopes have been synthesized by
organic chemists (Kaifu and Osawa, 1977; Ratcliffe et al.,
1981). T and Tn antigens are present on the external surface
of the cell plasma membranes of most CAs (Springer and Desai,
1977; Springer, 1984).

The observation of uncovered, autoimmunogenic T antigen on CA cell surfaces has opened a novel, promising ave-

nue in probing the specific interaction of a patient's immune system with his CA. CA patients mount strong humoral and cellular immune responses against at least one of these antigens. These responses are readily measurable in vivo and in vitro early and throughout the disease (Springer et al., 1976a; Springer and Desai, 1977; Springer et al., 1980; Thatcher et al., 1980; Vos and Brain, 1981; Bray et al., 1982, Bernhard et al., 1983).

The T antigen for measuring a person's immune response is readily obtained by removing sialic acid (NeuAc) from isolated erythrocyte membrane blood group MN glycoproteins of healthy donors (Springer and Ansell, 1958; Springer et al., 1966, 1976a).

T and Tn antigens have proved to be prominent histopathologic markers for all groups of CA tested (see e.g. Howard and Taylor, 1980; Boland et al., 1982; Coon et al., 1982; Ghazizadeh et al., 1984; Örntoft et al., 1985; Springer et al., 1985). Moreover, for some forms of CA, the densities of T and Tn on CA cells are histochemical predictors of the CA's invasiveness (Coon et al., 1982; Ghazizadeh et al., 1984; Springer et al., 1985). In addition, when present in the primary tumor, T and Tn were found in all metastases, as well as in tissue cell cultures derived therefrom, which points to the clonal nature of these markers (Springer, 1984; Springer et al., 1985).

We have shown in vitro that clusters of T and Tn epitopes are involved in the initial adhesion of some cancer cells to healthy epithelial tissue (Springer et al., 1983).

More than 25 laboratories throughout the world are currently working on T and Tn in relation to cancer. The predominant foci of these studies are a) immunohistochemical [even single breast CA cells were detected in local lymph nodes by virtue of their T antigen expression (Seitz et al., 1984)], b) measurement of specific anti-T autoantibody responses (Thatcher et al., 1980; Bray et al., 1982; Vos and Brain, 1981); and c) the location of cancer in vivo via its expression of T antigen (Shysh et al., 1985).

Here we present data on the importance of T and Tn autoantigens in breast CA, from both clinical and fundamental perspectives. We stress the apparent role of T and Tn in dynamic immunologic and nonimmunologic patient/breast CA interactions during the early phases of the disease.

MATERIALS AND METHODS

Test Subjects

Breast CA patients and controls were predominantly from the metropolitan Chicago area; most were Caucasian. In each cohort, all individuals were tested successively. We intended to measure cellular and humoral immune responses concomitantly, but this was frequently impossible. We fulfilled all institutional, U.S. National Cancer Institute, and U.S. Federal regulations concerning informed consent and ethical standards. Throughout, the results of only the initial test are listed. Patients were included only if there was no reasonable doubt as to the site of origin of the primary CA. We attempted to test the patients prior to biopsy, but succeeded in doing so only in the majority of Stage I patients. Among patients with incipient (Tis) breast CA, all but one were tested prior to biopsy. Patients who had received chemo- and/or radiotherapy were tested only after intervals deemed sufficient to obviate the gross interference of any therapy-induced change in immune response (cf. Springer, 1984). Tumor staging was postsurgical resection pathological throughout (Beahrs and Myers, 1983). All patients fully evaluated by a clinician-surgeon, pathologist, and by us are recorded here. The 142 breast CA patients studied include four males (one each Stage I and II infiltrating ductal and two Tis ductal).

Surgical Specimens

Malignant and control tissues for antibody absorption and neutralization were collected during surgery using the precautions and stringent controls previously described (Springer et al., 1980, 1985).

Cancer Cell Lines

Human cancer cell lines were grown in tissue culture. The nature of the cells, culture techniques, and the ascertaining of absence of mycoplasma and cytomegalovirus have

been described earlier, as has the nature and growth
of animal cancers as ascites tumors (Springer et al., 1985).

Cell-Mediated Immune Responses to T Antigen

   The delayed-type skin hypersensitivity reaction to T
antigen (DTHR-T). This test was performed on the upper,
outer arm contralateral to any putative or known breast lesion. T antigen preparation from MN glycoprotein isolated
from healthy human erythrocytes (RBC), testing procedures,
controls, interpretation, and absence of immunization by
the test itself, have been reported in detail (Springer et
al., 1966, 1976a, 1980). Briefly, T antigen was dissolved
at 1% final concentration in phosphate-buffered (pH 7.4)
physiological saline containing 0.25% phenol. The control
was solvent containing 1% MN antigen from which the particular batch of T antigen had been prepared. All reagents
and labware were sterile, free of pyrogens and HLA and he-
patitis B antigens. The solutions (0.1 ml each) were in-
jected intradermally (ID) 3.5 to 5 cm apart, using a Bec-
ton-Dickinson insulin syringe with a 28-gauge needle. All
subjects were also given one standard dose of mumps skin
test antigen (E. Lilly) and/or dermatophytin-O (Hollister-
Stier) as common antigen ID to ascertain the cell-mediated
immune competence of this predominantly tuberculin-negative
population.

   Induration and erythema were measured at about 24 hrs
after injection and again at 48 hrs unless the first read-
ing was clearly positive. The longest diameter of induration and the one perpendicular to it were averaged. Measurements were made independently by three investigators,
and averaged prior to interpretation; any reaction to MN antigen was subtracted from the corresponding reaction to T
antigen. An induration of $\geq$ 4 mm after 24 or 48 hrs was
considered a positive reaction (Springer et al., 1980).
There was one anergic individual among the Stage II and III
breast CA patients. She is not listed, since all her skin
reactions were negative.

   In vitro hemolytic autoimmune response of peripheral
blood lympho- and monocytes (PBLM) against erythrocytes expressing T antigen and control natural killer cell response.
We developed an assay that measures lysis of ^{51}Cr-labelled
autologous and homologous O RBC having maximally exposed (by

sialidase treatment) T antigen (T/RBC) as target cells, with
PBLM as effector cells (Robinson and Springer, 1984). The
PBLM of healthy persons show low-level lysis of such T/RBC.
The effect of PBLM on target T/RBC of breast disease patients, other patients, and healthy persons, and at least
one of the two healthy "standard" donors were tested in
parallel, correction for overall standard lysis was performed. Lysis was uniformly T/RBC-specific; RBC not treated
with sialidase were resistant to PBLM.

We assessed natural killer activity of the PBLM to
K 562 leukemia cells, in parallel with our hemolytic test,
using an established procedure (Fitzgerald et al., 1983).

T-specific inhibition of leukocyte migration (LMI) in
agarose. The principle of the assay was first described by
Clausen (1971). We have previously described the LMI test
of peripheral blood leukocytes, preincubated with T antigen
in agarose plates, including controls, standards and defi-
nition of positive and negative reactions (Springer et al.,
1980). We recently substituted Medium 199 for Hanks' bal-
anced salt solution, and now use 100 mm dishes rather than
60 mm dishes.

Humoral Responses to T Antigen

Blood was collected and separated as described (Springer et al., 1976a). The serum samples for determining anti-
T titer scores, anti-T globulin levels, and Ig measurement
were either worked up immediately or stored in small ali-
quots, at -80°C, earlier they were stored at -20°C, and re-
centrifuged immediately before use. Storage at these tem-
peratures prevents decay of anti-T antibodies (unpublished).

T/RBC were obtained after uncovering of T-specific receptors on O RBC by neuraminidase free of other glycosidases,
proteases and de-O-acetylases (Springer et al., 1972, 1976a).
Tn RBC were the generous gift of Drs. M. Beck and P. Lale-
zari. Preparations used consisted of ≥ 90% Tn RBC, either
fresh or preserved frozen in glycerol.

All hemagglutination and hemagglutination inhibition
assays in the determination of antibody specificity were
performed at least three times at ∿ 20°C, with controls and

standards as described earlier (Springer and Horton, 1969).
The volume of each reagent was 30 µl. A fresh pipette was
used for each titration step. All putative inhibitors used
have been described previously (Springer et al., 1983;
Springer and Desai, 1985). In the inhibition tests, 2 ag-
glutinating doses of antibody were used. The smallest quantity of putative inhibitor added that completely inhibited
agglutination was taken as the endpoint. Substances that
failed to inhibit hemagglutination at up to 90 µg were considered inactive. All readings were done by microscope, independently by three persons. Results were averaged.

Titrations of anti-T and -Tn antibodies were done by
routine blood banking procedures (Springer et al., 1976a).
In the assessment of anti-T titer scores the specificity of
the hemagglutination method is acceptable, but not its sensitivity. We therefore developed a solid-phase immunoassay
for sensitive and quantitative measurement of anti-T antibodies (SPIA-T) that has formed the basis of our humoral anti-T antibody studies since 1982. The principle of this
test, its controls, and standards have been described (Springer and Desai, 1982; Desai and Springer, 1984). SPIA-T uses T
antigen coupled to polyacrylamide beads in the quantitation
of serum anti-T Ig subclasses. Total serum Igs are determined in parallel, using commercially available reagents and
standards (Bio·Rad). We found the commercial standards also
to be valid as standards for our anti-T assays.

Anti-T antibodies consist predominantly of IgM, consti-
tuting 7-14% of total IgM, with some IgG and very little
IgA (Springer and Desai, 1982; Springer and Tegtmeyer, 1981).
Among breast CA patients total IgM concentration was within
the rather wide normal range. However, in most CA patients,
anti-T IgM, but not anti-T IgG, levels differed from those
of patients with other diseases and those of healthy persons, when related to the total IgM concentration in the
same specimen.

Sensitivity in detecting breast CAs was greatest when
the concentration of a person's anti-T IgM was related to
his total IgM by the value Q_M, calculated from the simple
formula $Q_M = [(\text{Anti-T IgM})^2/\text{Total IgM}] \times 100$. Q_M values
between 100 and 360 are considered normal. This range was
established using sera from healthy persons (Springer and
Desai, 1982; Desai and Springer, 1984).

Determination of T and Tn Antigens in Tissues

Semiquantitative or qualitative studies of these antigens were by tissue absorption, where the extent of antibody absorption, properly controlled, served as the measure
of antigen expression on the tissues (Springer et al., 1975,
1985); or by immunohistochemical tissue staining, where human polyclonal anti-T and anti-Tn were localized by sequential application of polyvalent rabbit anti-human immuno-
globulin, absorbed swine anti-rabbit immunoglobulin, and
peroxidase-anti-peroxidase reagent with appropriate chromogenic substrates. For rodent monoclonal antibodies, bio-
tinylated, affinity-purified horse anti-mouse IgG (H+L) was
used, followed by the addition of avidin-biotin-peroxidase
complex, and then the chromogenic substrate (cf. Springer
et al., 1985).

Monospecific Anti-T and -Tn Antibodies

Human polyclonal anti-T and -Tn antibodies were prepared by a modified Landsteiner-Miller procedure, as delineated (Springer and Horton, 1969); however, elution was at
48^OC. The same method was also used as an adjunct in specificity assessment of monoclonal antibodies.

For the preparation of monoclonal antibodies, DA rat
were immunized with group O erythrocytes on which T had
been maximally uncovered by neuraminidase, as described
earlier (cf. Springer, 1984). Spleen cells of immunized
rats were fused with Y3-Ag 1.2.3 rat myeloma cells. The
resulting hybridomas were grown in vitro as delineated by
others (Galfrè et al., 1979). We obtained anti-T and anti-Tn monoclonal antibodies as shown by hemagglutination,
hemagglutination-inhibition, and by absorption and elution
studies (Metcalfe et al., 1985).

Model to Study the Molecular Basis of Tumor Cell - Healthy
Tissue Interaction

Highly invasive and metastatic DBA/2 ESb murine lymphoma cells have more T- and Tn-specific epitopes on their
cell membranes than the parent Eb strain (Springer et al.,
1983), and only highly invasive ESb, but not the Eb, cells ad-
hered to syngeneic hepatocytes in a physiologic environment

(Schirrmacher et al., 1980). We therefore determined the specific inhibition of this adhesion with the putative inhibitors described (Springer et al., 1983), in the hope of learning about the molecular basis of this important interaction between tumor cell and normal cell.

RESULTS AND DISCUSSION

Cellular Autoimmune Responses of CA Patients to T Antigen

The results of the DTHR-T on all patients with breast disease, with other non-CA diseases, and on healthy controls are summarized in Table 1. DTHR-T was positive in 123 of 142 patients with ductal CA; i.e., the true positive ratio was 86.6. Remarkably, this figure includes a positive response in 24 of 28 patients (85.7%) with the earliest form (Tis) of ductal breast CA. It should be noted that ductal CA comprises nearly 90% of all breast CA and has the most ominous outlook.

Patients with lobular or tubular breast CA whose disease, at least initially, has a more favorable outlook than that of ductal CA (Fisher et al., 1975; DeVita et al., 1982), had a positive DTHR-T less frequently: 15 of 33 (45.5%) reacted positively. These two CA types together account for only about 10% of all breast CAs.

Of the 248 patients with benign breast disease, 228 had a negative DTHR-T (92% true negative ratio). Initially, 251 patients were classified by biopsy as having benign disease; 23 of these had a positive DTHR-T. The original slides of some with a reaction assumed to be falsely positive were sent to Dr. P.P. Rosen (Memorial Sloan-Kettering Institute), who found three to have in situ CA. Of the remaining 20 false positive cases, 18 had hyperplasia; in 14 of these it was atypically proliferative, i.e., premalignant (cf. Dupont and Page, 1985). Three still listed here as falsely positive subsequently developed breast CA.

Of the 19 patients who had cancers other than carcinomas, only the two with T lymphoma were positive. Patients with the following cancers reacted negatively (one of each): B-cell lymphoma; extrapulmonary carcinoid; astrocytoma; glioma; glioma-astrocytoma; liposarcoma; and leiomyosarcoma. Two

TABLE 1. Intradermal Delayed-Type Hypersensitivity Response
to Erythrocyte-Derived T Antigen (DTHR-T) at Initial Visit,
of Breast CA Patients and Controls; (pTNM Staging)

Category	DTHR-T Positive / Total Tested
Breast adenoCA	
Ductal	
Stage I, Tis	24/28
Stage I, infiltrating	25/30
Stage II and III[*]	56/66
Stage IV	18/18
Total	123/142
Lobular and tubular	
Stage I, in situ	7/10
Stage I, II & III infiltrating	8/23
Total	15/33
Benign breast disease[†]	20/248
Non-CA cancers[‡]	2/19
Noncancer diseases not related to breast	
Tumors	0/16
Other diseases [§]	2/118
Healthy	0/114

[*] Cancer tissues of seven negatively reacting patients test-
ed; two lacked T but had Tn.
[†] All but two of the 20 patients with positive DTHR-T had
hyperplasia, see text.
[‡] For description of non-CA cancers, see text.
[§] For description of the two positive patients, see text.
Their DTHR-T turned negative within 1 year.

patients with sarcomatous chordoma, two with pulmonary carcinoid, four with acute or chronic myelocytic leukemia, and
two with Hodgkin's disease in remission reacted negatively
(see Table 1). Table 1 also shows that two of 118 patients
with infectious, degenerative, or autoimmune diseases had a
positive DTHR-T; both were among the 17 patients with chronic
lung infections. Tissue of the lung lesion from one of the

positively reacting patients was available; it contained si-
alidase-producing β-hemolytic streptococci and had apparently
autochthonous unmasked T receptors (cf. Springer, 1984). We
have not found any positive DTHR-T among healthy, not recently
vaccinated individuals.

In Vitro Hemolytic Response to Autologous or Homologous T/
RBC

The PBLM from 26 of 45 (58%) ductal breast CA patients,
but only 1 of 8 (13%) with lobular CA, showed significantly
enhanced lysis of T/RBC relative to PBLMs of standard healthy
donors. Two of 25 (8%) patients with benign breast disease,
2 of 20 (10%) with various other benign diseases, and 4 of
41 (10%) healthy persons showed enhanced T/RBC lysis. Comparison of lysis by CA patients with that by patients with
benign diseases and that of healthy persons both give p values of <0.001 (Robinson and Springer, 1984). The lysis appears to be antibody-independent; homologous as well as hetero-
logous anti-T antibodies interfere with it. T/RBC lysis by
PBLM was independent of natural killer cell activity tested
in parallel using K 562 leukemia cells as targets (Robinson
and Springer, 1984).

Upon cell separation, lytic activity was retained by
sheep erythrocyte nonrosette-forming PBLM but not by rosette-
forming cytotoxic or cytotoxic plus helper T cells. Lytic
activity of PBLM from a given donor was increased at least
two- to four-fold in isolated adherent, monocyte-enriched
populations. Thus, T/RBC lysis, which is increased in most
patients who have breast CA-associated T antigen, and are
DTHR-T positive, may be due to monocyte-mediated cytotoxicity
directed to CA-associated T antigen (Robinson and Springer,
1985).

T-Specific In Vitro Inhibition of Leukocyte Migration (LMI)

Most breast CA patients studied by LMI also had a positive DTHR-T. At the initial visit 39 of 99 (39%) peripheral
blood leukocyte populations from breast CA patients had a
positive reaction; this figure includes 4 of 9 patients (44%)
with Tis ductal CA. The leukocytes of 11 of 25 patients
(44%) with lobular breast CA had a positive LMI reaction.
Leukocytes from 13 of 95 patients (14%) with benign breast

disease reacted positively and none of 29 healthy women (0%) did so.

Humoral Anti-T Response

Everyone has anti-T agglutinins, their level remains rather constant, except in liver cirrhosis (Friedenreich, 1930; Burnet and Anderson, 1947; Caselitz and Stein, 1953; cf. Boccardi et al., 1974). The anti-T and -Tn antibodies are elicited primarily by the intestinal flora (Springer and Tegtmeyer, 1981).

We were the first to note that this constancy of anti-body score does not apply to patients with breast and other CAs; a severe depression of anti-T was frequent, measurable even by our initially only semiquantitative scoring (Spring-er et al., 1976a; Springer and Desai, 1977). Forty of 189 breast CA patients (21.2%) had severely depressed anti-T titer scores $\leq$ 10 (normal score: 20-25), while in our in-itial study, only 14 of 270 (5.2%) patients with benign breast disease (mostly atypical, proliferative lesions) had such depressed anti-T titer scores (the percentage is still between 5 and 6% among >1,000 patients with benign breast disease tested as of June, 1985.) Among 200 non-CA patients without breast disease and among healthy individuals, there were three (1.5%) with scores $\leq$ 10 (one of whom developed breast CA within 6 months). These differences between CA pa-tients and the other populations are statistically significant (p < 0.001) (Springer et al., 1976a, 1978, 1979). Others have subsequently reported similar results (Luner et al., 1977; Thatcher et al., 1980; Vos and Brain, 1981; Bray et al., 1982). In $\sim$ 3% of breast CA an extraordinary increase of anti-T score to $\geq$30 suggests an immune response confined to IgM anti-T.

Not all "false positive" reactions in persons without histologic CA turned out to be false (Table 2). We followed 20 patients with "benign" breast disease but severely depressed anti-T for up to 8 years. Seven of these developed histologi-cally verified breast CA after the original nonmalignant diag-nosis. The remaining cases have as yet shown no sign of transi-tion to CA. The data in Table 2 are argument for surveillance of persons with depressed anti-T, but no histologic CA.

Surgery of the primary tumor led to a rebound or over-shoot of anti-T score in excess of 25% in 27 of 38 breast

TABLE 2. Severe Anti-T Agglutinin Alteration in 7 of 20 Patients Followed Longitudinally who were First Diagnosed by Histology Not to have Breast CA but who Subsequently Developed Histologically Verified Breast CA

Patient No.	Date of Breast Biopsy/Surgery and Diagnosis	Date Blood Obtained / Anti-T Agglutinin Score* (NORMAL RANGE: 20 to 25)					Date of Breast Biopsy/Surgery and Diagnosis	
383	9/3/74 Fibroadenoma	9/3/74 6	9/75 9	12/78 11		5/13/79 8	5/15/79 Infiltrating ductal CA, 6 cm Θ, anaplastic, 3/6 level 1, LN+, Stage III	5/21/80 14
394	9/6/74 Ductal-lobular proliferative hyperplasia	9/6/74 10	1/3/75 11			2/6/75 10	2/6/75 Intraductal CA, no CA in 30/30 LN, Stage I	5/18/79 17
1491 3/9/76 8	11/24/76 Ductal epithelial proliferative hyperplasia, fibrocystic disease						11/12/84 Infiltrating, poorly differentiated ductal CA. Metastasis to all 27 LN, Stage III	2/28/85 12
2546 12/8/75 21	5/77 Normal mammogram	10/78 14	12/80 12	1/83 15		12/28/83 14	12/28/83 Infiltrating ductal CA, Stage I	3/5/84 21
3026	11/12/79 Lobular & ductal hyperplasia, severe papillomatosis	11/12/79 14	5/22/80 14	3/17/81 13	4/1/82 12	8/16/85 8	8/16/85 Ductal CA, Stage III	
3065	8/23/79 Sclerosing angiogenic tumor	12/10/79 40	2/6/80 34	1/3/85 36	11/8/83 41	1/3/85 33	1/7/85 Infiltrating ductal CA, Stage I	
3072	9/16/76 Proliferative hyperplasia, fibrocystic disease	9/16/76 11				12/12/79 10	1/2/80 Lobular CA, Stage I	

* Indicative of CA: anti-T score ≤ 14 and ≥ 30 (the latter in absence of liver cirrhosis).

CA patients (71%) 1 to 5 months after surgery for the primary CA (see Table 2 for additional rebound data). Only one of 42 patients with biopsy and benign breast disease, and none of 22 who underwent non-CA surgery, responded similarly (p <0.001). This rebound implicates the CA as the cause of depressed anti-T, rather than a genetic defect that would render the patient unable to produce anti-T.

The SPIA-T quantitates anti-T Ig and overall Ig precisely and increases the sensitivity of early CA detection dramatically. It also surpasses standard commercial immune assays used for monitoring CA. For our findings on sera of patients with breast CA, benign breast disease, benign nonbreast diseases, and on healthy controls, see Table 3. CAs are categorized only according to stages because, in contrast to the DTHR-T, we found no notable difference between the various histological types. The humoral anti-T response of Tis breast CA patients is extraordinary; 23 of 27 reacted positively (true positive ratio, 85%). For all other CA stages combined, the true positive ratio is 80%. The second footnote in Table 3 lists all patients with benign breast disease; 94 of the 112 tested reacted negatively (true negative ratio, 84%). Two of 33 (6%) non-CA, nonbreast disease patients had a positive Q_M, as did 5 of 79 (6%) seemingly healthy persons (Table 3). Although ∿ 98% of all abnormal Q_M values in breast CA patients were depressed, the Q_Ms of two, one with Stage III breast CA (clinicopathologic: inflammatory CA) and one with Stage II [previously reported erroneously as Stage III (Springer, 1984)] were highly elevated (see first footnote, Table 3). This strong immune response was confined to anti-T IgM and may be indicative of a fundamental role of this anti-CA antibody in the pathogenesis of the disease. In one CA patient with strongly elevated anti-T Q_M, the DTHR-T could be determined and it was positive.-That not all benign disease or healthy persons with abnormal anti-T are "falsely positive" is indicated in Table 2.

Table 3 shows that 31 of 33 patients with benign nonbreast disease had a Q_M in the normal range; it was abnormal in two of 17 patients with chronic, infectious lung disease. Only the patient with an elevated Q_M had a positive DTHR-T. The likely reason, microbial uncovering of autochthonous T, for the false positive reactions has been discussed in the cellular immunity section.

TABLE 3. Anti-T IgM and Total IgM in Breast CA Patients and Controls, Measured at Initial Visit by Quantitative, Solid-phase Immunofluorescence Assay Values Expressed as the Quotient $Q_M = [(\text{Anti-T IgM})^2/\text{Total IgM}] \times 100$

| Category | Number of Subjects Tested* | Number with Q_M | | | Statistical Comparison of Q_M's of CA Patients, of Patients with Benign Diseases of the Same Organs, and of Healthy Persons | | | |
		De-pressed (< 100)	Nor-mal (100 to 360)	Ele-vated (> 360)	Mean	Stan-dard Devi-ation	95% Confi-dence Inter-val, and As-sertion of Difference Between CA and Benign	P Value for Ma-lignant Versus Benign
Breast CA (all types)								
Stage I, noninfil-trating (Tis)	27	23	4	0	68.6	26.8	26, 80	0.0000
Stage I, infiltra-ting	42	32	10	0	81.0	68.2	17, 66	0.0014
Stages II and III	38	31	7	0	85.1	68.0	3, 63	0.0017
Stage IV	4	4	0	0	54.7	14.8	41, 98	< 0.0025
Benign breast diseases†	38	6	32	0	125.1	37.9	62, 32	< 0.0015
Benign non-breast diseases	33	1	31	1	159.7	68.9	56, 115	0.0000
Healthy	79	5	74	0	171.0	77.1		0.0000‡

* Not listed are the results on the sera from two patients with Stages II and III ductal CA who had highly elevated Q_M's ($\bar{X}$ 463), see text. For details on abnormal Q_M's in patients with benign diseases, see text.

† We have now tested a total of 112 patients with benign breast disease; 94 had normal, and 18 had depressed Q_Ms. The true negative ratio (specificity) remains thus virtually unchanged. Neither detailed patho-histology nor statistics on these additional patients are as yet up to date.

‡ Compared to all CAs.

T and Tn Expression as Related to Carcinoma Aggressiveness

With Clive Taylor and colleagues, we have shown that
the relative proportions of T and Tn antigens on human
breast and other CAs frequently correlate with the CA's aggressiveness. More extensive studies in this area are in
progress with A. Klein-Szanto (to be published). In surgical specimens, the expression of T and Tn could be studied
in parallel. Of 15 well-differentiated breast CAs, 13 (87%)
had more T than Tn, whereas only 2 of 25 (8%) highly invasive, anaplastic primary breast CAs had more T than Tn. All
6 distant breast CA metastases tested had both T and Tn. T
also was expressed to a lesser degree than Tn in the few
poorly differentiated lung, pancreas, stomach, and colon CAs
investigated. This finding is consistent with the precursor
status of Tn vis-à-vis T (Springer and Desai, 1974, 1975;
Desai and Springer, 1979), but there are exceptions (Springer
et al., 1985).

Concomitantly we have shown in animal experiments that
there is a close correlation between density of T and Tn receptors on tumor cell surfaces and tumor invasiveness. In
two murine tumor lines—TA3 and Eb—live cells of a highly
invasive, metastatic subline were compared with those of the
minimally invasive parent. Both highly invasive sublines,
TA3-Ha and ESb, had more Tn than T on their outer cell surfaces; the parent lines had less of both antigens but more T
than Tn (Springer et al., 1985). All tissue culture and as-
cites-grown CAs tested, and also T lymphoblastic and stem
cells—but no other cell lines—had T and Tn activity (Springer et al., 1985). It is noteworthy that human DU 4475
secondary breast CA cells, when grown in Spinner culture for
prolonged periods, produce more Tn than T (Chandrasekaran,
E.V. and Springer, G.F., to be published). That T and Tn are
high up in the "pecking order" of CA antigens in primary as
well as metastatic CA is not only indicated by our studies of
these antigens, but also by our detection of five anti-T- or
anti-Tn specific monoclonal antibodies out of 13 raised
against CA tissue, which were kindly given to us by other investigators. Thus, in Table 4, the immunochemical specificity
of the anti-Tn from a pool of human A_1B donors (as stated
above, all humans have anti-Tn) is compared with monoclonal
anti-Tn prepared unwittingly by us using T/RBC, rat monoclonal T9 2c[A6] (Metcalfe et al., 1983, 1985; Springer and
Desai, 1985) and by Schlom, Colcher and colleagues, mouse
B 72.3 (Colcher et al., 1981) using human breast CA meta-

TABLE 4. Specific Inhibition of Tn Erythrocyte Agglutination by Anti-Tn Specific Antibodies

Putative Inhibitor	Mass (Da)	Monospecific Anti-Tn Antibodies					
		Human Polyclonal Pool La-Mi'84		Rat Monoclonal T9 2c[A6]		Mouse Monoclonal B 72.3	
		µg*	nmoles	µg	nmoles	µg	nmoles
AS-Glycoproteins -peptides†							
AS-OSM	620,000	1	0.002	3	0.005	3	0.005
T Antigen‡	555,000	45	0.081	90	0.162	45	0.081
Blood Group B Cyst Antigen	≈ 500,000	>90		>90		>90	
Tn Antigen Preparation (crude)§	39,000	9		18		15	
AS-Orosomucoid		>90		>90		>90	
AS-LS-α1 MN GP	12,000	30	2.5	30	2.5	30	2.5
AS-PII MN GP	7,000	30	4.3	30	4.3	30	4.3
Carbohydrates							
Me-α-GalNAc	235	4.5	19	3	12.8	3	12.8
p-Nitrophenyl-β-GalNAc	343	9	26	15	43.7	15	43.7
GalNAc	221	4.5	20.4	9	40.7	4.5	20.4
ManNAc	221	>90		90	407	>90	
Man	180	>90		90	500	>90	
GlcNAc	221	>90		>90		>90	
Gal	180	>90		>90		>90	
Galβ1→3GalNAc	383	>90		>90		>90	

* Smallest quantity completely inhibiting agglutination by two hemagglutinating doses, final vol 90 µl.

† Except for T antigen, whose mass was determined hydrodynamically (cf. Springer et al., 1979), calculated on the basis of molecular mass of parent compound and decrease due to NeuAc loss. The sialylated parent compounds were inactive. AS, asialo; OSM, ovine submaxillary mucin; AS-LS-α1 MN GP and AS-PII MN GP, defined cleavage products of T antigen. For more details on the nature of these compounds, see Springer et al. (1983).

‡ Derived from inactive MN blood type glycoprotein by desialylation.

§ Crude, inhomogeneous extract; its major component, Tn, corresponds to RBC-derived T glycoprotein but lacks most of its 13% Gal (Springer et al., 1979).

static tissue.

All three antibody preparations show characteristic anti-Tn specificity and are devoid of any other. Structures with multiple repetitive GalNAcα-O-Ser/Thr epitopes, preferably clustered as in asialo-ovine submaxillary mucin (AS-OSM), show extraordinarily high activities; $\leq$0.005 nmoles fully inhibit and the methyl α anomer of GalNAc is more active than the β form, having the highest activity of all haptens tested in accord with earlier studies (Springer and Desai, 1974; et al., 1975; Springer and Desai, 1975; Desai and Springer, 1979). All three antibodies listed in Table 4 were completely and specifically absorbable onto and extensively elutable from Tn RBC. Nevertheless, as would be expected, the specificity of the monoclonal reagents was somewhat more rigid than that of the human polyclonal anti-Tn antibody pool as shown in absorption studies with CA tissues (Springer et al., 1985).

Coon et al. (1982) demonstrated the predictive value of T antigen expression for future invasiveness of grades I and II papillomatous transitional-cell urinary bladder CAs. Immunohistochemical detection of an abnormal T antigen status in these tumors heralded a subsequent deep muscle invasion in more than 50%. For prostatic CA, a similar predictive value of T antigen expression in relation to invasiveness and metastasis has been recently reported by investigators in Japan (Ghazizadeh et al., 1984). Neither of these groups of authors has yet reported on the CA-associated Tn antigen in these malignancies.

The data presented show that anti-T and anti-Tn are anti-CA antibodies shared by everyone, and that immunoreactive T and Tn are associated with about 90% of all CA but are not accessible in other tissues.

The relationship between CA aggressiveness and expression of T and Tn epitopes in absolute terms and relative to one another prompted us to investigate whether the role of T and Tn was confined to immunologic patient — tumor interaction. Our experiments with an animal model system in vitro indicate that the expression of T and Tn antigens on CA cells has profound pathogenic and clinical consequences. Clusters of T and Tn epitopes on cancer cell membranes appear to be cell adhesion molecules, binding to healthy tissues (Fig. 1) in at least the primary step of CA invasion which is adhesion.

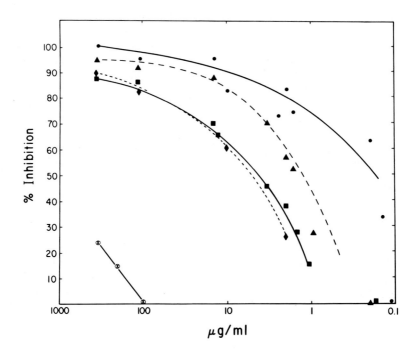

Figure 1. Inhibition in vitro of murine ESb T lymphoma cell adhesion to syngeneic hepatocytes by T- and Tn-active AS-glycoproteins and -glycopeptides (AS-LS-GP). OSM was the source of the Tn-specific macromolecule. Symbols: ●─────●, AS-LS-α1 MM GP; ▲─ ─ ─ ─ ▲, T antigen (MN blood group-derived); ■─────■, AS-LS-α1 NN GP; ◆- - - - - -◆, AS-OSM; ⊗─────⊗, Galactopyranosyl-β-1→3-N-acetyl-D-galactosamine.

Attachment of the ESb cancer cells, whose membranes are rich in T and Tn epitopes, to hepatocytes was competitively inhibited by minute quantities of T antigen and by AS-OSM (Springer et al., 1983), which we had shown earlier to be highly Tn-active (Springer and Desai, 1974). AS-OSM's carbohydrate moiety is almost exclusively composed of Gal-NAc-α-O-Ser/Thr clusters. The effect of the inhibitors was

specific; their sialylated parent compounds and other structures with different asialo-heterosaccharides (not shown in
Fig. 1) had little or no activity.

Products of T glycoprotein cleavage that possess T-ac-
tive heterosaccharide clusters were most active in the adhesion inhibition assay, and the potency of inhibition increased with the extent of clustering per peptide chain; the
free T hapten, Galβl→3GalNAc, had only trace activity
(Springer et al., 1983).

CODA

The basis for the unique presence of T- and Tn-immuno-
reactive structures in CAs is unknown. T and Tn, as already
indicated, may be stage-specific fetal differentiation antigens (Springer et al., 1984). As indicated above, T and
Tn are distributed three-dimensionally over the entire cell-
surface glycoconjugate coat of CA. They may be directly involved in the temporal processes of invasion and uncontrol-
led growth. Perhaps the CA cell membrane has a causative
role in both processes, and regulating it may control CA.
CA adhesion may initiate feedback to further proliferation
and invasion.

Incipient CAs may have a gradual local redistribution
of negative charges by altered sialylation, coupled with con-
formational changes at the outer cell membrane. This may
be a key factor in allowing the CA to attach itself to
healthy cells via the uncovered T- and Tn-specific structures. These changes, however, may not satisfy the free
energy requirements for interaction with cellular and humoral anti-T components of the immune system. It would be
a narrow view to consider only one mechanism for the survival and establishment of CA cells in vivo. Nevertheless,
the "sneaking through" hypothesis is supported by studies
in vitro (Springer and Desai, 1982).

To the best of our knowledge, two of our assays that
use T antigen (DTHR-T and SPIA-T) are the only ones that detect breast CA at its earliest stages (see Tables 1 and 3),
and with great reliability. Earliest possible detection of
breast CA is mandatory. This view has been recently under-
scored by the finding that of 17 patients in whom nonpal-
pable preclinical breast CA in situ was diagnosed by mammo-

graphy, <u>all</u> developed clinical breast CA within 4 to 37
months (Stark, 1985).

ACKNOWLEDGMENT

The authors thank Prof. M. Dwass for his help with
the statistics, Drs. J. Schlom and D. Colcher for mouse monoclonal antibody B 72.3 and permission to publish our findings
with it, and Prof. W.T.J. Morgan, F.R.S. for human blood
group B cyst glycoprotein. This work was supported by NCI
Grants CA 19083, CA 22540 and the Elsa U. Pardee Foundation.

REFERENCES

Beahrs OH, Myers MH (eds) (1983). "Manual for Staging of Cancer," 2nd ed., Philadelphia: JB Lippincott, pp 6-9, 127-133.
Bernhard MI, Wanebo HJ, Helm J, Pace RC, Kaiser DL (1983).
Leukocyte migration inhibition responses to MCF-7, murine
mammary tumor virus, and Thomsen-Friedenreich antigen in
a series of cancer patients. Cancer Res 43:1932-1937.
Boccardi V, Attinà D, Girelli G (1974). Influence of orally
administered antibiotics on anti-T agglutinin of normal
subjects and of cirrhotic patients. Vox Sang 27:268-272.
Boland CR, Montgomery CK, Kim YS (1982). Alterations in
human colonic mucin occurring with cellular differentiation
and malignant transformation. Proc Natl Acad Sci USA 79:
2051-2055.
Bray J, Maclean GD, Dusel FJ, McPherson TA (1982). Decreased
levels of circulating lytic anti-T in the serum of patients
with metastatic gastrointestinal cancer: a correlation with
disease burden. Clin Exp Immunol 47:176-182.
Burnet FM, Anderson SG (1947). The "T" antigen of guinea-pig
and human red cells. Aust J Exp Biol Med Sci 25:213-217.
Cartron JP, Andreu G, Cartron J, Bird GWG, Salmon C, Gerbal
A (1978). Demonstration of T-transferase deficiency in Tn-
polyagglutinable blood samples. Eur J Biochem 92:111-119.
Caselitz FH, Stein G (1953). Experimentelle Beiträge zum
Problem der Hämagglutination nach Thomsen. Z ImmunForsch
exp Ther 110:165-184.
Clausen JE (1971). Tuberculin-induced migration inhibition
of human peripheral leucocytes in agarose medium. Acta
Allergol 26:56-80.
Colcher D, Hand PH, Nuti M, Schlom J (1981). A spectrum of
monoclonal antibodies reactive with human mammary tumor

cells. Proc Natl Acad Sci USA 78:3199-3203.

Coon J, Weinstein RS, Summers J (1982). Blood group precursor T antigen expression in human urinary bladder carcinoma. Am J Clin Pathol 77:692-699.

Dahr W, Uhlenbruck G, Gunson HH, Hart Mvd (1975). Molecular basis of Tn-polyagglutinability. Vox Sang 29:36-50.

Dausset J, Moullec J, Bernard J (1959). Acquired hemolytic anemia with polyagglutinability of red blood cells due to a new factor present in normal human serum (anti-Tn). Blood 14:1079-1093.

Desai PR, Springer GF (1979). Biosynthesis of blood group T-, N-, and M-specific immunodeterminants on human erythrocyte antigens. J Immunogenet 6:403-417.

Desai PR, Springer GF (1980). Sialylation of Thomsen-Friedenreich (T) and type NM antigens by transferases in human sera measured by $[^{14}C]$NAN uptake. J Immunogenet 7: 149-155.

Desai P, Springer G (1984). Carcinoma detection by quantitation and interrelation of serum anti-T IgM and total IgM. In Peeters H (ed): "Protides of the Biological Fluids," Vol. 31, New York: Pergamon Press, pp 421-424.

DeVita VJ, Hellman S, Rosenberg SA (eds) (1982). "Cancer Principles and Practice." Philadelphia: JB Lippincott.

Dupont WD, Page DL (1985). Risk factors for breast cancer in women with proliferative breast disease. New Eng J Med 312:146-151.

Fisher ER, Gregorio RM, Fisher B, Redmond C, Vellios F, Sommers SC, cooperating investigators (1975). The pathology of invasive breast cancer. A syllabus derived from findings of the National Surgical Adjuvant Breast Project (Protocol No. 4). Cancer 36:1-85.

Fitzgerald PA, Evans R, Kirkpatrick D, Lopez C (1983). Heterogeneity of human NK cells: comparison of effectors that lyse HSV-1-infected fibroblasts and K562 erythroleukemia targets. J Immunol 139:1663-1667.

Friedenreich V (1930). "The Thomsen Hemagglutination Phenomenon." Copenhagen: Levin and Munksgaard.

Galfrè G, Milstein C, Wright B (1979). Rat x rat hybrid myelomas and a monoclonal anti-Fd portion of mouse IgG. Nature 277:131-133.

Ghazizadeh M, Kagawa S, Izumi K, Kurokawa K (1984). Immunohistochemical localization of blood group precursor T-antigen in benign hyperplasia and adenocarcinoma of the prostate. J Urol 132:1127-1130.

Howard DR, Taylor CR (1980). An antitumor antibody in normal human serum: reaction of anti-T with breast carcinoma cells. Oncology 37:142-148.

Kaifu R, Osawa T (1977). Synthesis of O-(2-acetamido-2-deoxy-α-D-galactopyranosol)-N-tosyl-L-serine. Carbohydr Res 58:235-239.

Lloyd KO, Kabat EA (1968). Immunochemical studies on blood groups. XLI. Proposed structures for the carbohydrate portions of blood group A, B, H, Lewis[a] and Lewis[b] substances. Proc Natl Acad Sci USA 61:1470-1477.

Luner SJ, Wile AG, Sparks FC (1977). Antibody to T and Tn antigens in patients with breast cancer. Proc Amer Assoc Cancer Res, Abstract No. 375.

Metcalfe S, Springer GF, Svvennsen RJ, Tegtmeyer H (1985). Monoclonal antibodies specific for human Thomsen-Friedenreich (T) and Tn blood group precursor antigens. In Peeters H (ed): "Protides of the Biological Fluids," Vol. 32, Oxford: Pergamon Press, pp 765-768.

Metcalfe S, Svvennsen RJ, Springer GF, Tegtmeyer H (1983). Monoclonal antibodies to tumour associated Thomsen-Friedenreich (T) and Tn antigens. J Immunol Methods 62:M8.

Örntoft TF, Mors NPO, Eriksen G, Jacobsen NO, Poulsen HS (1985). Comparative immunoperoxidase demonstration of T-antigens in human colorectal carcinomas and morphologically abnormal mucosa. Cancer Res 45:447-452.

Ratcliffe RM, Baker DA, Lemieux RU (1981). Synthesis of the T [β-D-Gal-(1→3)-α-D-GalNAc]-antigenic determinant in a form useful for the presentation of an effective artificial antigen and the corresponding immunoadsorbent. Carbohydr Res 93:35-41.

Robinson MK, Springer GF (1984). Cellular hemolytic autoimmune response of carcinoma patients against erythrocytes expressing T antigen. Proc Amer Assoc Cancer Res 25:280.

Robinson MK, Springer GF (1985). Role of monocytes in carcinoma patients' lytic immune response to erythrocytes expressing T antigen. Proc Amer Assoc Cancer Res 26:317.

Schirrmacher V, Cheingsong-Popov R, Arnheiter H (1980. Hepatocyte-tumor cell interaction in vitro. J Exp Med 151: 984-989.

Seitz RC, Fischer K, Stegner HE, Poschmann A (1984). Detection of metastatic breast carcinoma cells by immunofluorescent demonstration of Thomsen-Friedenreich antigen. Cancer 54:830-836.

Shysh A, Eu SM, Noujaim AA, Suresh MR, Longenecker BM (1985). Radioimmunodetection of murine mammary adenocarcinoma (TA3/Ha) lung and liver metastases with radioiodinated PNA. Int J Cancer 35:113-119.

Springer GF (1984). T and Tn, general carcinoma autoantigens. Science 224:1198-1206.

Springer GF, Ansell NJ (1958). Inactivation of human erythrocyte agglutinogens M and N by influenza viruses and receptor-destroying enzyme. Proc Natl Acad Sci USA 44:182-189.

Springer GF, Cheingsong-Popov R, Schirrmacher V, Desai PR, Tegtmeyer H (1983). Proposed molecular basis of murine tumor cell - hepatocyte interaction. J Biol Chem 258:5702-5706.

Springer GF, Desai PR (1974). Common precursors of human blood group MN specificities. Biochem Biophys Res Commun 61:470-475.

Springer GF, Desai PR (1975). Human blood-group MN and precursor specificities: structural and biological aspects. Carbohydr Res 40:183-192.

Springer GF, Desai PR (1977). Cross-reacting carcinoma-associated antigens with blood group and precursor specificities. Transplant Proc 9:1105-1111.

Springer GF, Desai PR (1982). Detection of lung- and breast carcinoma by quantitating serum anti-T IgM levels with a sensitive solid-phase immunoassay. Naturwissenschaften 69:346-348.

Springer GF, Desai PR (1985). Tn epitopes, immunoreactive with ordinary anti-Tn antibodies, on normal, desialylated human erythrocytes and on T (Thomsen-Friedenreich) antigen isolated therefrom. Molecular Immunol, in press.

Springer GF, Desai PR, Banatwala I (1974). Blood group MN specific substances and precursors in normal and malignant human breast tissue. Naturwissenschaften 61:457-458.

Springer GF, Desai PR, Banatwala I (1975). Blood group MN antigens and precursors in normal and malignant human breast glandular tissue. J Natl Cancer Inst 54:335-339.

Springer GF, Desai PR, Murthy MS, Scanlon EF (1978). Human carcinoma-associated precursors of the blood group MN antigens. In Walborg E (ed): "Symp Glycoproteins and Glycolipids in Disease Processes." Washington: Amer Chemical Society, pp 311-325.

Springer GF, Desai PR, Murthy MS, Tegtmeyer H, Scanlon EF (1979). Human carcinoma-associated precursor antigens of the blood group MN system and the host's immune response to them. In Kallós P, Waksman BH, deWeck AL, Ishizaka K (eds): "Progress in Allergy," Vol. 29, Basel: S Karger, pp 42-96.

Springer GF, Desai PR, Scanlon EF (1976a). Blood group MN precursors as human breast carcinoma-associated antigens and "naturally" occurring human cytotoxins against them. Cancer 37:169-176.

Springer GF, Desai PR, Schachter H, Narasimhan S (1976b). Enzymatic synthesis of human blood group M-, N- and T-specific structures. Naturwissenschaften 63:488-489.

Springer GF, Desai PR, Tegtmeyer H, Schirrmacher V, Cheing-song-Popov R (1983). Murine lymphoma cells possess blood group Tn-, T-, N-, M- and S-active substances. Naturwissenschaften 70:98-99.

Springer GF, Horton RE (1969). Blood-group isoantibody stimulation in man by feeding blood group-active bacteria. J Clin Invest 48:1280-1291.

Springer GF, Murthy MS, Desai PR, Scanlon EF (1980. Breast cancer patient's cell-mediated immune response to Thomsen-Friedenreich (T) antigen. Cancer 45:2949-2954.

Springer GF, Nagai Y, Tegtmeyer H (1966). Isolation and properties of human blood-group NN and meconium-Vg antigens. Biochemistry 5:3254-3272.

Springer GF, Taylor CR, Howard DR, Tegtmeyer H, Desai PR, Murthy SM, Felder B, Scanlon EF (1985). Tn, a carcinoma-associated antigen, reacts with anti-Tn of normal human sera. Cancer 55:561-569.

Springer GF, Tegtmeyer H (1981). Origin of anti-Thomsen-Friedenreich (T) and Tn agglutinins in man and in White Leghorn chicks. Br J Haematol 47:453-460.

Springer GF, Tegtmeyer H, Cromer DW (1984). Are T and Tn differentiation antigens? Fed Proc 43:6.

Springer GF, Tegtmeyer H, Huprikar SV (1972). Anti-T reagents in elucidation of the genetical basis of human blood-group MN specificities. Vox Sang 22:325-343.

Stark AM (1985). Screening for breast cancer. Lancet 1: 1102.

Thatcher N, Hashmi K, Chang J, Swindell R, Crowther D (1980). Anti-T antibody in malignant melanoma patients. Cancer 46:1378-1382.

Vos GH, Brain P (1981). Heterophile antibodies, immunoglobulin levels, and the evaluation of anti-T activity in cancer patients and controls. S Afr Med J 60:133-136.

Tumor Markers and Their Significance in the Management
of Breast Cancer, pages 71–88
© 1986 Alan R. Liss, Inc.

Monoclonal Antibody Characterization of a Tumor-associated
Breast Cancer Antigen[1]

Dean P. Edwards, Lynn G. Dressler, David T. Zava
and William L. McGuire

University of Colorado Health Sciences Center
Department of Pathology,
Denver, Colorado 80262[2]

INTRODUCTION

Monoclonal antibodies (MAb's) reactive with breast
cancer-associated antigens have been developed recently by
several investigators. These antibodies fall into two
general categories. There are those directed against
antigens which are highly restricted to breast cancer
(Colcher et al. 1981; Nuti et al. 1982; Cardiff et al. 1983;
Soule et al. 1983; White et al. 1985) and not expressed on
normal cell counterparts. These antibodies are potentially
useful in diagnosis and therapy of breast cancer since they
can distinguish between breast tumor cells and normal
breast. Another group of MAb's have been raised against
tissue differentiation antigens of normal breast epithelium. These normal breast epithelial antigens are also
expressed, although in reduced amounts, on a majority of
breast carcinomas and are potentially useful as well in
diagnosis of breast cancer (Papsidero et al. 1983; Croghan
et al. 1983; Menard et al. 1983; Canevari et al. 1983;
Mariani-Costantini et al. 1984; Taylor-Papadimitriou et al.
1981; Arklie et al. 1981; Ceriani et al. 1977, 1981, 1983;
Burchell et al. 1983).

[1] Supported by National Institutes of Health Grants CA-30195,
HD-10202 and Robert A. Welch Foundation.

[2] (DTZ): John Muir Aging & Cancer Institute, Walnut Creek,
CA 94596; (LGD and WLM): Univ of Texas Health Sciences
Center, Department of Medicine, San Antonio, TX 78284.

We have produced a MAb against MCF-7 human breast
cancer cells which is of the first category since it recognizes an antigen expressed predominantly on breast carcinoma
and is not found in most normal human tissues. This paper
describes properties of this MAb which includes immunohistochemical evaluation of in vivo tissue distribution of antibody binding and biochemical characterization of the antigen
recognized by this monoclonal antibody.

Screening Strategy and Production of MAb's

Mice were immunized by injection with 1×10^7 live
MCF-7 cells given i.p. once a week for 3 weeks. Animals
were boosted 3 days before fusion with a 3 M KCl extract of
purified MCF-7 membrane vesicles. Spleen cells were removed
and fused with mouse NS-1 myeloma using 50% polyethylene
glycol as the fusion agent. Cell fusions, propagation of
hybrid cells in HAT selection medium and subcloning have
been previously described in detail (Edwards et al. 1984).

Since our goal was to define antigens that might serve
as tumor markers in breast cancer, our screening strategy
was designed to select monoclonal antibodies reactive with
surface membrane antigens highly restricted to breast cancer
cells and not expressed on normal tissue counterparts.

Screening of hybridomas was performed in several
stages, each stage designed to eliminate unwanted MAb's.
(1) The first level of screening was by enzyme linked
immunosorbent assay (ELISA) against a panel of methanol
fixed tissue culture cell lines. This panel included breast
cancer cell lines, non-breast human cell lines, animal cell
lines, and HBL-100 which is derived from normal human milk
epithelium. Only those antibodies showing high binding to
breast cancer lines and low or no binding to other cells
were taken for cloning and further analysis. (2) Since we
were interested in MAb's against surface membrane antigens
positives were screened secondarily by an indirect immuno-
fluorescence assay with viable and lightly fixed MCF-7 cells
to assess whether antigens are localized on the surface of
cells. Antibodies reactive with intracellular structures
were eliminated and only those giving surface membrane
fluorescence staining were retained. (3) Antibodies were
further selected for their ability to recognize antigen in
paraffin embedded sections. To accomplish this, MCF-7 cells

were fixed in Bouin's solution, embedded in paraffin, thin sections were cut and the sections were stained by the avidin-biotin immunoperoxidase method (Ciocca et al. 1982). (4) Antibodies meeting all the above criteria were evaluated for immunoperoxidase staining with a limited number of formalin-fixed paraffin sections of breast carcinomas and normal human tissues, including normal breast. Those reactive with breast carcinomas but failing to react with normal tissues were taken for more extensive immunohisto-chemical and biochemical studies. Others were dropped from the study.

Approximately 3,000 hybridomas were screened by the above strategy and one particular MAb, designated 323/A3, has proven to be the most specific for breast cancer. The 323/A3 MAb is a mouse IgG$_1$ and the hybridoma cells secreting the 323/A3 MAb have been subcloned repeatedly and found to be a stable antibody producing line. The cells have also been successfully frozen in liquid nitrogen and regrown without loss of antibody production. The 323/A3 hybridoma cell line was grown as an ascites tumor in Balb/c mice and the IgG fraction was purified from ascites fluid by ammonium sulfate precipitation and DEAE-cellulose chromatography which yields approximately 95% purity of IgG. This fraction was used in all subsequent characterization studies.

Binding of 323/A3 to Cultured Cell Lines

A fixed-cell ELISA assay according to the method of Layton and Smithyman (1983) was used, with some modifica-tions, for assessment of 323/A3 binding to cell lines. Briefly, cells were plated in 96-well microtiter culture dishes at a density of 5×10^4 cells/well and allowed to grow for 24 h to form an attached monolayer. Cells were rinsed in phosphate buffered saline (PBS), dried by heating at 37°C for 30 min and, fixed for 5 min at room temperature with 70% methanol containing 3% hydrogen peroxide. Un-reactive sites were blocked by incubation with 1% bovine serum albumin (BSA) and cells were incubated overnight at 4°C with the MAb followed by a 3 h incubation at room temperature with goat anti-mouse IgG-peroxidase. Enzyme reaction and further details of the ELISA assay are to be published elsewhere. The following cell lines were examined for 323/A3 binding: MCF-7, MDA-231, ZR75-1, MDA-330, T47D, BT-20 (human breast cancer); HBL-100 (derived from normal human milk epithelium); KB (human oral epidermoid cancer); WI-38 (transformed human lung fibroblast); Balb/3T3 (mouse embryo fibroblast--clone A31); CHO (Chinese hamster ovary).

As shown in Figure 1, strong binding was obtained with four (MCF-7, T47-D, ZR-75.1, and BT-20) of the 6 human breast cancer cell lines assayed when using a single concentration of MAb. MCF-7, T47-D, and ZR-75.1 are steroid receptor positive cells, while BT-20, MDA-231 and MDA-330 are receptor negative (Horwitz et al. 1978; Engel, Young 1978). The ELISA data, therefore, suggest a lack of relationship between steroid receptors and expression of 323/A3 antigen in breast cancer. Little or no binding of the 323/A3 MAb was obtained with the non-breast cancer cell lines examined, including HBL-100 which is derived from normal human breast epithelium.

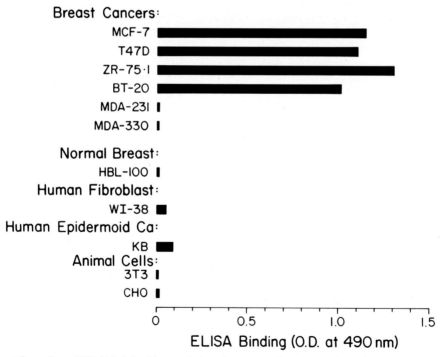

Fig. 1. 323/A3 binding with tissue culture cell lines as measured by fixed cell ELISA. (Further details to be published in Cancer Research.)

Figure 2 shows titration of 323/A3 binding, by fixed cell ELISA, to MCF-7 cells compared with other antigen negative cell lines. Antibody source was highly purified 323/A3 MAb from mouse ascites fluids. MAb concentrations ranged from 10 μg/ml to 750 pg/ml. At the highest concentrations of 323/A3 no binding above background was obtained with any of the non-breast cancer cell lines. By contrast half-maximal binding of 323/A3 with MCF-7 cells occurs at about 10 ng/ml of MAb with the end point dilution occurring at below 750 pg/ml. Thus, antigen densities on MCF-7 are orders of magnitude higher than on these other cell lines. Similar ELISA binding dose curves were observed with the other antigen positive breast cancer cells (data not shown).

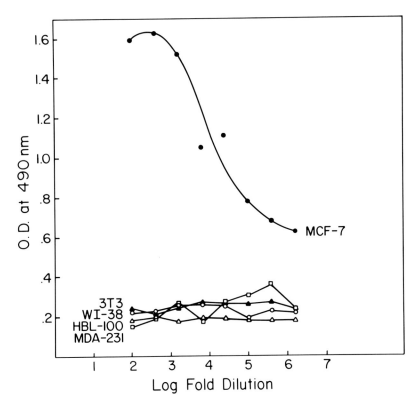

Fig. 2. Titration of 323/A3 binding to methanol fixed cell cultures by ELISA assay. (To be published in further detail in Cancer Research.)

Immunohistochemical Studies with 323/A3 MAb

To determine the intracellular localization of the
antigen recognized by the 323/A3 MAb, indirect immuno-
fluorescence (IF) assays were performed with both live and
lightly fixed MCF-7 cells. With lightly fixed cells grown
on chamber slides a fairly even fluorescent staining of cell
membranes and a diffuse weak staining of cytoplasm was
observed with the 323/A3 MAb. On the other hand, a granular
fluorescent staining was observed on the surface of viable
unfixed cells in suspension indicating surface localization
of the 323/A3 antigen (not shown). Surface membrane localization was also indicated by 323/A3 MAb binding by ELISA to
detergent and 3 M KCl extracts of purified MCF-7 plasma
membranes. Moreover, immunoperoxidase staining of paraffin
sections of MCF-7 cell pellets is also predominantly
membrane. Thus, the 323/A3 antigen appears to be localized
on the surface of MCF-7 cells and is stable to fixation and
embedding in paraffin.

The ability of the 323/A3 MAb to detect antigen in
paraffin sections has allowed us to use formalin-fixed
paraffin sections of human tissues for our immunocytochemical studies. This is an advantage since it allowed us
to obtain a greater variety and number of tissues that might
otherwise have been inaccessible in other forms (i.e., fresh
frozen sections). Immunocytochemistry was performed as
previously described (Ciocca et al. 1982) using the avidin-
biotin-peroxidase complex (ABC) to evaluate in vivo tissue
distribution of 323/A3 binding.

The results of 323/A3 immunoperoxidase staining of
formalin-fixed paraffin sections of human breast tissues are
summarized in Table 1. Normal breast, benign tumors, and
malignant lesions of the breast were examined. No staining
was observed with normal breast, which included two cases of
lactating breast and eight resting breast. Of the benign
tumors examined, 20% showed binding with 323/A3. The
immunostaining of benign tissues was heterogeneous and was
localized primarily to surface membranes in areas of epithelial cell hyperplasia and apocrine glands. Histologically normal lobules and stroma do not stain. The incidence
of 323/A3 reactivity in benign tumors increased with the
degree of epithelial cell hyperplasia and was particularly
intense in histologically "high risk" tissue sections containing intraductal or lobular hyperplasia with atypia.

Table 1

323/A3 Immunoperoxidase Staining of Human Breast Tissues[1]

Tissue	No. positives/ No. of tissues tested	% positive	Location of stain
Normal breast	0/10	0	-
Benign breast disease	13/63	20	m,c[2]
Breast carcinoma	76/128	59	m,c
Metastatic nodes	6/8	75	m,c

[1] A section was considered positive if greater than 1% of cells stained with the 323/A3 MAb.
[2] c = cytoplasm, m = membrane (adapted from Mansel et al., to be published elsewhere)

These preliminary findings with benign tumors suggests that expression of the 323/A3 antigen may increase with progression of breast disease. Of the primary breast carcinomas examined, 59% reacted with 323/A3 and, although the number of cases are low, a slightly higher percentage of metastatic lymph nodes stained positively (Table 1). Thus, the incidence of immunocytochemical staining with 323/A3 was observed to increase in a progressive manner from normal, to benign disease, to metastatic lesions suggesting that the 323/A3 antigen may be a marker of disease progression and possibly of pre-malignancy.

Among the 76 positive breast carcinomas examined the pattern of 323/A3 immunoperoxidase staining was highly heterogeneous. For example, the percentage of immunostained tumor cells within a given tumor ranged from 1 to 100% (mean = 58%) and intensity of staining ranged on an arbitrary scale from +1 to +4. Intracellular location of staining was also highly heterogeneous. Some tumors showed predominantly cytoplasmic staining (45%), others predominantly membrane staining (11%) while the majority (54%) gave both cytoplasmic and membrane staining. In no case did we observe 323/A3 staining of blood vessels, surrounding connective tissues or with morphologically normal breast epithelium adjacent to tumor cell involvement. In metastatic

lymph nodes only tumor cells were stained. No staining was
observed with normal lymphocytes. Antibody reactivity in
breast tumors, therefore, was confined to neoplastic epithelial cells with the exception that staining was associated
in some tumor sections with hyperplastic epithelial cells
and apocrine glands in areas adjacent to tumor cell
involvement.

We have also examined the immunocytochemical reactivity
of 323/A3 with some non-breast human tumors. Binding was
observed with several other adenocarcinomas, including endometrial, colon, thyroid and prostate carcinomas and, in each
case, immunostaining was confined to involved epithelial
cells. As with breast carcinoma staining was localized to
both membranes and cytoplasm. Although we have examined
only a few cases, 323/A3 has not shown reactivity, so far,
with tumors of non-epithelial origin. The antibody
therefore does not react exclusively with breast carcinomas,
but binds also with other cancers of epithelial origin.

In order to evaluate in vivo tissue distribution, we
further examined binding of 323/A3 by immunoperoxidase (ABC)
with a large variety of normal human tissues. 323/A3 did
not bind with the vast majority of tissues examined, including normal breast, spleen, pancreas, heart, lung, liver,
prostate, ovary, endometrium, thyroid, small intestine,
skeletal muscle, stomach, lymph nodes, skin, bone marrow,
and blood vessels. The only exceptions on this list of
normal human tissues are positive reactions observed with 2
of 8 kidneys and 5 of 5 colons. Staining of kidney was weak
and localized to collecting tubules and was not observed in
glomerulus or capillary systems. All five cases of colon
examined gave a positive heterogeneous staining localized to
surface epithelium and intestinal glands. Goblet cells do
not stain and binding appears to be localized to the basal
region of surface and glandular epithelial cells.

Based on our immunocytochemical analysis, the 323/A3 MAb
appears to bind with a high degree of selectivity to mammary
and other carcinomas but not with the vast majority of
normal human tissues examined, including normal breast.
Since 323/A3 reacts solely with epithelial elements (whether
tumor or normal cells), it may be recognizing a normal
epithelial surface antigen expressed in abnormally high
concentrations in tumors of epithelial origin.

Characterization of 323/A3 Antigen

Immunoblot analysis was used initially to define the
structure of the antigen recognized by 323/A3. Immunoblots
(Western blots) were performed essentially as described by
Towbin et al. (1979). Briefly, cell and membrane protein
extracts were resolved on SDS-polyacrylamide electrophoresis
gels as described by Laemmli (1971), the resolved proteins
were electrophoretically transferred to nitrocellulose
filters and then reacted with the 323/A3 MAb followed by an
^{125}I-labeled second antibody (goat anti-mouse IgG). Immunoreactive protein bands were detected by autoradiography.
MCF-7 and human breast tumor plasma membrane vesicles were
isolated by centrifugation of cell extracts on discontinuous
sucrose density gradients as described by Riordan and Ling
(1979). In initial experiments NP-40 extracts of purified
MCF-7 membranes were analyzed by immunoblotting and no
immunoreactive bands were detected. Subsequently we
examined the conditions for preservation of antigenicity by
a dot blot assay in which MCF-7 membrane extracts were
spotted onto nitrocellulose discs and incubated with the
323/A3 MAb followed by an ^{125}I-labeled second antibody and
counting of the filter disc for radioactivity. Heating to
100°C or denaturation with various detergents, including 1%
SDS, did not affect 323/A3 binding to antigen. However,
treatment with reducing agents such as β-mercaptoethanol
destroyed all antigenic activity. Western blots, therefore,
were repeated using an electrophoresis SDS-sample buffer
both with and without β-mercaptoethanol and results are
shown in Figure 3. Also included in Figure 3 is a 323/A3
Western blot analysis with membrane extracts from MDA-231
cells which by ELISA were negative for the 323/A3 antigen.
In the presence of β-mercaptoethanol no immunoreactive bands
were detected in either MDA or MCF-7 cell extracts.
However, in the absence of reducing agent a single immunoreactive band was detected in MCF-7 membranes at M_r =
43,000 which was absent in MDA cells. In this experiment,
decreasing amounts of MCF-7 membrane extracts were used
ranging from 95 to 12 μg of total protein.

Immunoprecipitation studies were performed with MCF-7
proteins metabolically labeled in culture with [^{3}H]glucos-
amine. Radiolabeled cell extracts were incubated with 323/
A3 and then immunoabsorbed with a rabbit antimouse second
antibody and Protein-A-Sepharose beads. After washing, the
Protein-A-beads were extracted with SDS-sample buffer and

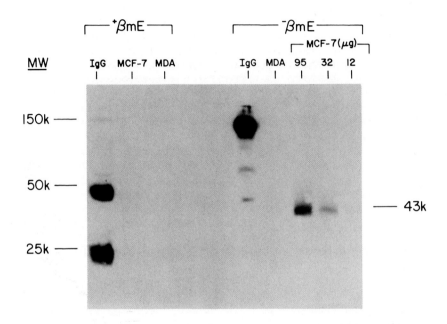

Fig. 3. Western blot analysis of detergent membrane extracts from MDA-231 and MCF-7 human breast cancer cells with 323/A3 MAb. Membrane extracts were dissolved in SDS-sample buffers with β-mercaptoethanol (+βME) and without β-mercaptoethanol (-βME). ^{125}I-IgG is a molecular weight marker. (Further details to be published in Cancer Research.)

the extracts were analyzed by SDS-gel electrophoresis and scintillation counting of gel slices. A single radioactive peak was detected at M_r = 43,000, whereas no radioactive peak was obtained by incubation with negative control NS-1 ascites fluid (not shown; details to be published in Cancer Research). Both reducing and non-reducing gels of the same radiolabeled immunoprecipitates gave single M_r = 43,000 radioactive peaks, indicating that the antigen is not likely to be associated with a larger multimeric complex which reduces to M_r = 43,000 subunits, but is simply sensitive to reducing agent.

The glycoprotein nature of the antigen was further characterized by determining lectin binding specificities.

Membrane extracts of MCF-7 cells were dialyzed against 10 mM Hepes buffer, pH 7.2, containing 0.15 M NaCl and 0.1% NP-40, and passed over various lectin-agarose affinity columns equilibrated in the same buffer. The columns were washed extensively and then eluted with specific sugars and the column fractions were analyzed for the presence of 323/A3 antigen by Western blot. The 323/A3 antigen appeared to display the following order of binding affinities for lectins; ulex europeaus > Con A > wheat germ > and no binding was observed with lens culinaris and ricinus communis I. Specific elution of the M_r = 43,000 antigen from Con A columns was obtained with α-methylmannoside (not shown).

To determine whether the 323/A3 MAb was recognizing the same antigen in human tumors in vivo as in MCF-7 cells, Western blots were also performed with plasma membranes isolated from a pool of frozen human breast tumors and compared with MCF-7 membranes. The 323/A3 MAb reacts with a single M_r = 43,000 band in membranes of actual human tumors which co-migrates with the M_r = 43,000 antigen detected in MCF-7 membranes. Thus antigen in tumors in vivo appears to be the same protein as that detected in MCF-7 cell cultures.

DISCUSSION

By use of monoclonal antibody technology we have identified an antigen which is expressed predominantly on breast cancer and is not found on most normal tissues examined including normal breast. The antigen recognized by the 323/A3 MAb is a 43,000 dalton glycoprotein which appears to be the same protein in MCF-7 cells and in breast tumors in vivo. As yet we do not know if the determinants recognized by the MAb are carried on the carbohydrate or the polypeptide portion of the antigen. Preliminary tunicamycin inhibition experiments suggest that the MAb binds with protein but that carbohydrate may also be important for its binding affinity. As with many other tumor-associated antigens, the 323/A3 antigen appears to be a surface membrane protein and represents only a minor component of the cell surface. Surface binding of the 323/A3 MAb is indicated by live-cell (MCF-7) immunofluorescence binding assays. Also supportive of surface membrane localization is the fact that the M_r = 43,000 antigen is contained only in isolated plasma membrane vesicles of subfractionated MCF-7

cells and is not found in soluble cytoplasm. Our more
recent finding that the antigen is released in significant
amounts into the medium of MCF-7 cultures (unpublished data)
is also indicative of surface localization. In human breast
tumor sections assayed by immunoperoxidase procedures,
staining was associated with both cytoplasm and membrane.
Since tissues were fixed with formalin, intracellular
antigen localization is difficult to interpret by these
immunoperoxidase staining assays.

Only a handful of MAb's have been produced by other
investigators which recognize breast cancer-associated antigens that are not also present on normal breast epithelium
or widely distributed on other normal human tissues (Cardiff
et al. 1983; Soule et al. 1983; White et al. 1985; Horan-
Hand et al. 1983). The 43,000 dalton glycoprotein identified in our studies is distinct from these other breast
tumor-associated antigens either in molecular weight or in
tissue distribution determined by immunocytochemistry.
Based on comparison of molecular weights (for those antigens
which have been chemically characterized) the 323/A3 antigen
is also distinct from tumor-associated antigens detected by
MAb's in other tumor systems including antigens associated
with melanoma, brain tumors, colorectal, ovarian, lung and
renal carcinomas as well as leukemias and lymphomas (see
review by Lloyd,(1983). There is also no similarity
between the 323/A3 antigen and the CA antigen recently
described by Ashall et al. (1982). CA is an antigen
expressed on a majority of tumors (primarily of epithelial
origin), which is found in very few normal tissues and is a
two component membrane glycoprotein of M_r = 350,000 and
380,000 believed to be correlated with malignancy of a
tumor. The 323/A3 antigen is also distinct from carcinoembryonic antigen (CEA) in molecular weight and in tissue
distribution,based on immunocytochemistry studies of others
with antibodies to CEA (Colcher et al. 1983). We were also
unable to block binding of 323/A3 MAb to MCF-7 cells with
purified CEA.

Studies by other investigators have for the most part
resulted in production of MAb's that are directed against
breast cancer determinants that are also expressed on normal
mammary epithelium. Some have been produced through
immunization with breast cancer cell lines (Papsidero et
al. 1983; Croghan et al. 1983; Menard et al. 1983; Canevari
et al. 1983; Mariani-Costantini et al. 1984) and others by

immunization with human milk fat globule membranes (Taylor-Papadimitriou et al., 1981; Ceriani et al. 1977, 1981, 1983; Arklie et al. 1981; Burchell, 1983). The 323/A3 MAb appears also to be distinct from this class of antibodies since we observe no reactivity with normal breast epithelium and very limited binding with other normal tissues. The 323/A3 MAb, therefore, appears to recognize a previously undescribed breast tumor-associated antigen and thus adds to the small repertoire of MAb's available which can distinguish between normal and neoplastic breast cancer cells.

The ability of our MAb to detect antigen in paraffin sections of surgical specimens is of particular advantage, since this has allowed us to screen a large number of tissues rather rapidly by immunoperoxidase methods. It will also allow us to perform retrospective studies. As has been the case with other tumor-associated antigens described in the literature, we found after rigorous examination of many tissues by immunohistochemistry that the 323/A3 antigen is not absolutely tumor specific nor is it disease specific. Although reactivity of 323/A3 MAb with normal human tissues is very limited, we have observed binding with all normal colons examined and weak staining with two sections of renal tubules. Otherwise, examination of multiple cases of a large variety of tissues reveals that the 323/A3 antigen is either absent or below the level of detection in all other normal human tissues. The M_r = 43,000 glycoprotein, therefore, is a tumor-associated antigen in the sense that normal breast contains no detectable level of antigen whereas it is expressed in a majority of breast carcinomas. In normal colon the 323/A3 antigen is localized solely to epithelial cells and binding observed so far with tumors of different histologic types are all tumors of epithelial origin. The 323/A3 antigen, therefore, may represent a normal colon epithelial antigen also expressed on tumors of epithelial origin and antigen expression on these different tumor types may be occurring through a common mechanism.

Because of its high specificity for breast cancer (as well as benign breast lesions) and cell surface localization, the 323/A3 antigen may be an important biological marker in breast cancer and the MAb against the antigen may have potential application in both diagnosis and treatment of breast cancer. Since the 323/A3 antigen can be detected in paraffin sections, it may be a useful biochemical marker for immunohistochemical identification of breast tumor cells. There are situations for example in which mammary dysplasia, distant metastasis and pleural effusions are difficult to diagnose morphologically. The MAb may also be useful in localization of tumor metastasis by external body radioimaging techniques. Although the 323/A3 antigen is present in some benign breast lesions and in normal colon, absolute specificity is not necessary for successful radio-localization of tumors. What is required is a sufficient differential in antigen concentration to be able to achieve good contrast between tumors and surrounding normal tissues. The most promising potential, however, may be the use of this MAb in early screening of breast cancer. Towards this end we may be able to apply 323/A3 in two ways. First, our immunohistochemical studies with a large series of benign breast disease specimens indicates that 323/A3 may be identifying those benign lesions which, based on morphological criterion, are believed to be at high risk to development of malignancy. For example, the highest frequency of positive staining was observed with lesions of the greatest epithelial hyperplasia and morphological dysplasia. The 323/A3 antigen, therefore, may be a potentially important biochemical marker in benign breast disease. Both prospective and retrospective studies are now being done to examine the relationship between antigen expression and risk to develop cancer. Measurement of shed 323/A3 antigen in serum may prove to be a second method of early breast cancer screening. Since antigen is not detected in most normal tissues and our preliminary data show release of antigen by MCF-7 cells into culture medium, it may be present in detectable amounts in human serum at very early stages of breast cancer and not present in normal serum. We do not know yet if antigen present in normal colon will complicate or preclude the development of a serum screening assay. We do not know, for instance, whether the immunoperoxidase staining observed with normal colon is due to the presence of the 43,000 dalton glycoprotein or whether it represents cross reaction with other determinants. Nor do we know whether antigen in colon is also a surface protein and able to be released. Finally, the 323/A3 MAb may be of potential therapeutic value. Since the antibody does not react with normal bone marrow,it may be very effective as an antibody-toxin conjugate in eliminating breast cancer cells in vitro from bone marrow for use in autologous marrow transplantation. As recently reported by LeMaistre et al. (1985),the 323/A3 MAb conjugated with the

A-chain of ricin was found to be a very potent and highly selective cytotoxic agent for breast cancer cells in vitro.

All these potential applications, however, must be considered in the context that the 323/A3 antigen is expressed in about 60% of breast tumors in vivo. Since this MAb by itself will not detect all breast tumors in vivo, it will be necessary to develop additional MAb's with characteristics similar to 323/A3, but directed toward different antigens, so that a mixture of MAb's can be put together that will detect the other 40% of breast tumors. It may also be important in the future to combine the 323/A3 MAb with other presently available MAb's in order to achieve detection of 100% of breast tumors.

Arklie J, Taylor-Papadimitriou J, Bodner W, Egan M, Millis R (1981). Differentiation antigens expressed by epithelial cells in the lactating breast are also detectable in breast cancers. Int J Cancer 28:23-29.

Ashall F, Bramwell ME, Harris H (1982). A new marker for human cancer cells. 1. The Ca antigen and the CA_1 antibody. Lancet July 3:1-6.

Burchell J, Durbin H, Taylor-Papadimitriou J (1983). Complexity of expression of antigenic determinants recognized by monoclonal antibodies HmFG-1 and HmFG-2, in normal and malignant human mammary epithelial cells. J Immunol 131:508-513.

Canevari S, Fossati G, Balsari A, Sonnino S, Colnaghi MI (1983). Immunochemical analysis of the determinants recognized by a monoclonal antibody (mBr-1) which specifically binds to human mammary epithelial cells. Cancer Res 43:1301-1306.

Cardiff RD, Taylor CR, Wellings SR, Colcher D, Schlom J (1983). Monoclonal antibodies in immunoenzyme studies of breast cancer. Ann NY Acad Sci 420:140-146.

Ceriani RL, Thompson K, Peterson JA, Abrahams S (1977). Surface differentiation antigens of human mammary epithelial cells carried on the human milk fat globule. Proc Natl Acad Sci USA 74:582-586.

Ceriani RL, Orthendahl D, Sasaki M, Kaufman L, Miller S, Wara WM, Peterson JA (1981). Use of human mammary epithelial antigens (HME-Ags) in breast cancer diagnosis. Cancer Detect Preven 4:603-609.

Ceriani RL, Peterson JA, Lee JY, Moncada R, Blank EW
(1983). Characterization of cell surface antigens of
human mammary epithelial cells with monoclonal antibodies
prepared against human milk fat globule. Somatic Cell
Genet 9:415-427.
Ciocca DR, Adams DJ, Bjercke RJ, Edwards DP, McGuire, WL
(1982). Immunohistochemical detection of an estrogen
regulated protein by monoclonal antibodies. Cancer Res
42:4256-4258.
Colcher D, Horan-Hand P, Nuti M, Schlom, J (1981). A
spectrum of monoclonal antibodies reactive with human
mammary tumor cells. Proc Natl Acad Sci USA 78:3199-3203.
Colcher D, Horan-Hand P, Nuti M, Schlom J. Differential
binding to human mammary and nonmammary tumors of monoclonal antibodies reactive with carcinoembryonic antigen.
Cancer Invest 1:127-138.
Croghan GA, Papsidero LD, Valenzuela LA, Nemoto T,
Penetrante R, Chu TM (1983). Tissue distribution of an
epithelial and tumor-associated antigen recognized by
monoclonal antibody F36/22. Cancer Res 43:4980-4988.
Edwards DP, Weigel NL, Schrader WT, O'Malley BW, McGuire WL
(1984). Structural analysis of chicken oviduct progesterone receptor using monoclonal antibodies to the subunit B
protein. Biochemistry 23:4427-4435.
Edwards DP, Gryzb KT, Dressler LG, Zava DT, Mansel RE,
McGuire WL (submitted). Monoclonal antibody identification and characterization of a 43,000 dalton membrane
glycoprotein associated with human breast cancer. Cancer
Res.
Engel LW, Young NA (1978). Human breast carcinoma cells in
continuous culture: A review. Cancer Res 38:4327-4339.
Horan-Hand P, Nuti M, Colcher D, Schlom J (1983). Defini-
tion of antigenic heterogeneity and modulation among human
mammary carcinoma cell populations using monoclonal
antibodies to tumor-associated antigens. Cancer Res
43:728-735.
Horwitz KB, Zava DT, Thilagar AK, Jensen EM, McGuire WL
(1978). Steroid receptor analysis of nine human breast
cancer cell lines. Cancer Res 38:2434-2437.
Kufe DW, Nadler L, Sargent L, Shapiro H, Horan-Hand P,
Austin F, Colcher D, Schlom J (1983). Biological behavior
of human breast carcinoma-associated antigens expressed
during cellular proliferation. Cancer Res 43:851-857.
Laemmli UK (1971). Cleavage of structural proteins during
the assembly of a head bacteriophage T4. Nature
227:680-685.

Layton GT, Smithyman AM (1983). A cell ELISA technique. The direct detection and semi-quantitation of immuno-globulin positive cells in 7 day lymphocyte cultures using the microtitre culture plates as solid phase. J Immunol Methods 57:37-42.

LeMaistre CF, Edwards DP, Dressler LG, Lathan B, Mansel RE, McGuire WL (1985). Studies with monoclonal antibodies to breast cancer. In Ceriani RL (ed): "Proceedings of International Workshop on Monoclonal Antibodies and Breast Cancer," Boston: Martinus Nijhoff Publishers (in press).

Lloyd KO (1983). Human tumor antigens: Detection and characterization with monoclonal antibodies. In Herberman RB (ed): "Basic and Clinical Tumor Immunology," Boston: Martinus Nijhoff Publishers, pp 159-214.

Mariani-Costantini R, Colnaghi MI, Leoni F, Menard S, Cerasoli S, Rilke F (1984). Immunohistochemical reactivity of a monoclonal antibody prepared against human breast carcinoma. Virchows Arch [Pathol Anat] 402:389-404.

Menard S, Tagliabue E, Canevari S, Fossati G, Colnaghi MI (1983). Generation of monoclonal antibodies reacting with normal and cancer cells of human breast. Cancer Res 43:1295-1300.

Nuti M, Teramoto YA, Marianni-Costantini R, Horan-Hand P, Colcher D, Schlom J (1982). A monoclonal antibody (B72.3) defines patterns of distribution of a novel tumor-associated antigen in human mammary carcinoma cell populations. Int J Cancer 29:539-545.

Papsidero LD, Croghan GA, O'Connell MJ, Valenzuela LA, Nemoto T, Chu TM (1983). Monoclonal antibodies (F36/22 and M7/105) to human breast carcinoma. Cancer Res 43:1741-1747.

Riordan JR, Ling, V (1979). Purification of P-glycoprotein from plasma membrane vesicles of Chinese hamster ovary cell mutants with reduced colchicine permeability. J Biol Chem 254:12701-12705.

Soule HR, Linder E, Edgington TS (1983). Membrane 126-kilodalton phosphoglycoprotein associated with human carcinomas identified by a hybridoma antibody to mammary carcinoma cells. Proc Natl Acad Sci USA 80:1332-1336.

Taylor-Papadimitriou J, Peterson JA, Arklie J, Burchell J, Ceriani RL, Bodmer WF (1981). Monoclonal antibodies to epithelium-specific components of the human milk fat globule membrane: Production and reaction with cells in culture. Int J Cancer 28:17-21.

Towbin H, Staehelin T, Garclam J (1979). Electrophoretic transfer of proteins from polyacrylamide to nitrocellulose sheets. Proc Natl Acad Sci USA 76:4350-4354.

White CA, Dulbecco R, Allen R, Bowman M, Armstrong B (1985). Two monoclonal antibodies selective for human mammary carcinoma. Cancer Res 45:1337-1343.

III. Estrogen Metabolites and Estrogen-Induced Proteins

Tumor Markers and Their Significance in the Management
of Breast Cancer, pages 91–103
© 1986 Alan R. Liss, Inc.

BIOCHEMICAL EPIDEMIOLOGY OF BREAST CANCER

Jack Fishman, Richard J. Hershcopf and
H. Leon Bradlow
The Rockefeller University
1230 York Avenue
New York, NY   10021

In the United States, and this is largely true of
the world in general, about one out of eleven women will
develop breast cancer in her lifetime. Abundant evidence
exists that this incidence is not random but that factors
exist which enhance the risk of developing this disease.
Epidemiological evidence dating back to the observations
of Beatson of the beneficial effect of oophorectomy in
breast cancer (Beatson, 1886); provides a strong argument
that endogenous estrogens play a role in the etiology and
progress of human breast cancer and that they are involved
in one or more of the risk factors. Because of this, much
effort has been directed to the identification of
differences in the secretion and/or metabolism of
estrogens in women with breast cancer but the results
obtained have so far been contradictory and the existence
of such differences remains in question (Zumoff et al,
1975).

In retrospect, the absence of significant
differences in the estrogenic patterns in breast cancer
patients is not surprising. The development of breast
cancer is a slow process with the initiation of the
disease apparently taking place many years before overt
symptoms appear. In the so called "window" hypothesis of
breast cancer inception (Korenmann, 1980), there are
specific periods of increased vulnerability to such
initiation in the early post pubertal years and again in
the perimenopausal period. For example, studies of
survivors of the Hiroshima bomb show that those exposed to
the radiation during their teens show the greatest
incidence of breast cancer 20 - 30 years later.

The protective effect of a first pregnancy prior to age 25 also indicates that hormonal changes in this early age period (MacMahon et al, 1970) influence the appearance of the disease in postmenopausal years. Similarly, oophorectomy is protective of later development of breast cancer only if carried out prior to 30 years of age (Trichopoulas et al, 1972). The many studies of estrogen secretion and metabolism in postmenopausal breast cancer patients offer no information about the endocrine milieu at the time when the disease was initiated and hence may not provide insights into the role of estrogen secretion or metabolism as a risk factor for breast cancer. We therefore sought to find a measure of estrogen metabolism which is not affected by age or menopausal status and which when measured in the postmenopausal women would reflect her metabolic profile at the time of disease initiation.

The metabolism of estradiol (Fig. 1) is almost exclusively oxidative in nature, involving a series of hydroxylations and oxidations which are briefly described below. Estradiol (E_2), the primary glandular secretory product, is first oxidized to estrone (E_1) (Fishman et al, 1960), followed by a series of reversible conjugations and irreversible hydroxylations leading to, among others, 16-hydroxyestrone and 2-hydroxyestrone (Fishman et al, 1980). Estrone is the linch pin of this combination of reactions and the principal precursor for the irreversible reactions. The 16α-hydroxylative pathway leads to 16α-hydroxyestrone and then estriol. The alternative hydroxylation at C-2 yields the catechol estrogens, principally 2-hydroxyestrone, which have been found to have both estrogen agonist and antagonist properties, and whose biology appears to be distinct from the parent hormone (Martucci and Fishman, 1977).

Two principal methods can be employed to evaluate the metabolic transformation of estrogens. The classical approach involves the intravenous administration of a radiolabeled estrogen and the analysis of the radiolabeled metabolites in urine and blood samples obtained after the injection (Hellman et al, 1967). The procedure is complex and labor intensive. There are significant manipulative losses but most importantly urinary excretion is variable and accounts for only 50-70% of the administered radioactivity with no information being provided about the

Table 1

Oxidation of Estradiol at C-2,16, and 17
in Normal Men and Women

Subjects	Age	% Dose oxidized, mean ± SD		
		2-Hydroxylation	16-Hydroxylation	17-Oxidation
Men	23-62	20.8±7.6(19)*	7.5±1.9(19)^	62.9±10.5(20)>
Premenopausal Women	27-35	38.9±1.2(6)*	10.7±2.1(7)<^	83.8±15.4(6)>
Postmenopausal Women	48-70	32.6±1.3(7)	8.5±1.4(9)<	73.7±18.5(6)

Numbers in ( ) represent numbers of subjects
* P < 0.001
^ P < 0.005
\> P < 0.005
< P < 0.025

4-HYDROXYESTRADIOL   4-HYDROXYESTRONE   ESTRADIOL   ESTETROL

2-METHOXYESTRONE   2-HYDROXYESTRONE   ESTRONE   16α-HYDROXYESTRONE

2-METHOXYESTRADIOL   2-HYDROXYESTRADIOL   2-HYDROXYESTRIOL   ESTRIOL

missing elements (Zumoff et al, 1968). Studies of
hormonal changes in cancer patients can also be affected
by non-specific illness effects which can significantly
alter enterohepatic circulation and urinary metabolic
patterns (Zumoff et al, 1971). The alternative
radiometric procedure involves the administration of a
precursor, labeled with tritium at a metabolically
reactive site, from which the tritium is transfered to
body water upon oxidation or hydroxylation at that
position (Fishman et al, 1980). The extent of reaction is
followed by measuring the tritium specific activity of
water derived from blood and urine samples collected at
intervals over 24-72 hours. This technique has the
advantage that the total extent of a particular reaction
can be obtained without the need to isolate or
characterize any metabolites and without concern for
further transformations or excretory routes. Its
disadvantage resides in that the method provides no
information regarding conjugative or further metabolic
steps. As we have described, the rate and extent of the
principal oxidative transformations of estradiol at C-2,
16α and 17 sites permits their studies to be carried out
sequentially and allows the generation of total profile of
these reactions in 5 days (Fishman et al, 1980). Since 2-
and 16α -hydroxylation are largely mutually exclusive,
they can be ascertained individually with little concern
for the existence of dual transformations in the same
molecule.

    In our studies of estradiol metabolism in normal
pre- and postmenopausal women using this radiometric
procedure, we have established that the activity of the
three enzymes varies little with age (Fishman et al, 1980)
(Table 1), and that the metabolic pattern determined in a
postmenopausal woman should reflect that existent in her
reproductive years. Examining the extent of the three
oxidative transformations of estradiol in post- and
perimenopausal women with breast cancer and matched
controls (Schneider et al, 1982), we found that there is a
highly significant increase in the extent of 16 α-
hydroxylation in the cancer patients compared to the
controls, but that the other two transformations are not
different (Table 2). As can be seen from the results in
Fig. 2 there is little overlap between the breast cancer
population and the control group with respect to a 16 α-
hydroxylation. We conclude, therefore, that unless the

Table 2

Maximal Percentage of Oxidation of [2-^{3}H]estradiol

[16α-^{3}H]estradiol, and [17α-^{3}H]estradiol in vivo*

	Estradiol Metabolism[a], % Oxidation		
Subjects	2-Hydroxylation	16α-Hydroxylation	17-Oxidation
Breast Cancer Women	32.7 ± 2.7(25)	14.9 ± 1.5(15)	73.0 ± 4.2(13)
Normal Women	31.1 ± 4.0(10)	9.3 ± 0.8(10)	76.9 ± 5.3(10)
P	NS	< 0.01	NS

NS - not significant
*In breast cancer patients and normal controls
[a] Mean ± SEM, the number of subjects studied is in parentheses

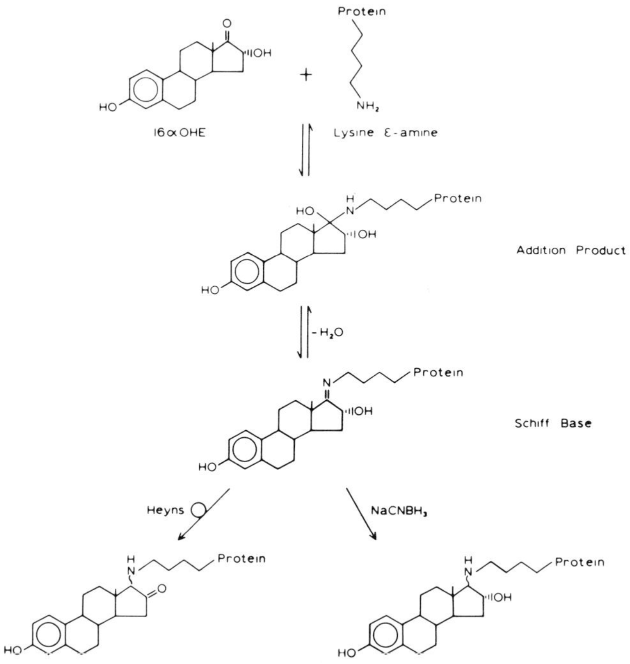

Figure 2. Maximal 16 α-^{3}H-estradiol oxidation in 10 control women and in 15 patients with breast cancer. Values expressed are ^{3}H$_2$O formed as a percentage of the administered dose. Means are represented by horizontal dashed lines.

process is disease induced, the increased 16α -
hydroxylation found in older women with cancer was most
probably present in the earlier premenopausal years of
their life.

Evidence that this elevated metabolic reaction is a
pre-existing risk marker for the disease, and is not the
result of the mammary tumor, is derived from our studies
of 16α -hydroxylation in several mouse strains with widely
different incidence of spontaneous breast tumors.
Measurement of the reaction in 6-8 week old mice from
different strains employing a modification of the
radiometric procedure used in the human studies showed
that the extent of 16α -hydroxylation of estradiol is
positively correlated with the incidence of tumor
formation (Bradlow et al). Since these experiments were
carried out well before the age at which spontaneous
tumors appear the increased 16α -hydroxylation in these
mice was present prior to the onset of overt disease.
These measurements were highly reproducible when
individual strains of mice were restudied at 3-6 month
intervals and the differences between different strains
were highly significant statistically. If the estrogen
component of the disease in the mouse model is in any way
related to human breast cancer, these observations suggest
that increased 16α -hydroxylation of estrogens may also be
a risk factor in human breast cancer. This animal model,
therefore, if verified, provides an important means of
studying the role of this transformation in the etiology
of mammary tumors.

The only other human disease in which we have
observed a consistent elevation in 16α -hydroxylation of
estrogens is in systemic lupus erythematosus (SLE) a
disease which is predominant in women (Lahita et al,
1979). However, unlike breast cancer, in SLE the increase
in 16α -hydroxylation is accompanied by a concomitant
decrease in 2-hydroxylation of the hormone suggesting that
different metabolic defects are involved in these two
diseases.

The two products of the 16α -hydroxylative pathway
are 16α -hydroxyestrone and estriol and the question
remains whether the increase 16α -hydroxylase activity
results in an increased formation of one or the other or
in both of these metabolites. In the case of the SLE

patients the principal 16α-hydroxylation product which is increased is 16 α-hydroxyestrone and not estriol (Lahita et al, 1981). Reexamination of previously obtained data in breast cancer patients in which biologically stable labled estradiol was administered also showed that formation of 16α-hydroxyesterone and not estriol was increased in these subjects. At this time, however, we have as yet not measured 16α-hydroxylase activity and urinary metabolic profile in the same subjects to establish that such a relationship exists. The indications are however that 16 α-hydroxyestrone is the metabolite principally increased by the elevated activity of this enzyme and the biological properties of this estrogen become of acute interest. While the pharmacology and physiology of estriol has been extensively studied that of 16 α-hydroxyestrone has largely been ignored.

Estriol has been the subject of considerable controversy for many years concerning its possible role as an estrogen antagonist in breast cancer. Because the compound showed an apparently limited estrogenic response in animal tests (Huggins and Jensen, 1957) and because of the belief that the protective effect of early pregnancy was due to estriol, several investigators proposed that the administration of estriol might exert a protective action against breast cancer (Lemon, 1972). In fact, urinary estriol in breast cancer patients has been reported in various studies to be either elevated (Hellman et al, 1971) or depressed (Lemon et al, 1966) relative to control subject. In an attempt to buttress the estriol hypothesis it was subsequently proposed that the critical determinant is not the absolute level of estriol (E3) but the ratio or excreted E3/(E1 + E2) between menarche and menopause (MacMahon et al, 1973). When the concept was tested by comparing the ratio in low risk Japanese women versus high risk British (Bulbrook et al, 1976) or American women (MacMahon et al, 1974) conflicting results were obtained, with the U.S. study showing a highly significant difference in estriol ratios while the British study showed no difference. Critical examination of the U.S. study showed, however, that estriol was actually identical in the two populations, with all of the differences concentrated in the denominator ($E_1 + E_2$) (MacMahon et al, 1973). More recently MacMahon and colleagues, in a similar study comparing women with early pregnancies (<age 25) and those with later pregnancies,

found a highly significant difference in the $E_3/(E_1 + E_2)$ between the two groups (Cole et al, 1976), with the difference concentrated in the estriol component. Subsequently, however, these same investigators have cast doubt on the estriol hypothesis (MacMahon et al, 1982).

The possible protective effect of estriol has also been challenged in animal studies. When estriol was tested under physiological conditions with continuous administration it was found to be fully uterotrophic (Clark et al, 1977). In addition, estriol, when administered continuously, induced mammary tumors in rats (Rudali et al, 1975, Poortman, 1980). The net balance of all these findings is that estriol is an estrogen agonist under physiological conditions. Increased 16 α-hydroxylation need not be reflected only in increased formation of estriol, but in an excess of the initial product of the reaction, 16 α-hydroxyestrone (16α OHE_1) and this appears to be the case in breast cancer. Thus 16 -hydroxylation needs to be considered both in terms of its initial product, 16 OHE_1 a potent and possibly unique estrogen agonist, and its further metabolite, estriol, which appears to behave as a conventional estrogen agonist under physiological conditions (Hilgar, 1968). That increased formation of 16α -hydroxyestrone can have significant biological consequences is indicated by an examination of its properties. Although it has only a very modest affinity for the estrogen receptor it appears to be fully equivalent to estradiol as an estrogen agonist in several test systems (Martucci and Fishman, 1977). In addition it has full biological availability in the human since it does not bind to SHBG, the principal estrogen binding protein in plasma (Martucci and Fishman, 1977). Most importantly, it is unique among all of the estrogens, of being able to form nonenzymatically covalent bonds with the primary amino groups of biological macromolecules (Bucala et al, 1984). These adducts occur via a stabilized Schiff base formation followed by a thermodynamically favored Heyn's rearrangement (Fig. 3). Such interactions have now been demonstrated to occur in vitro and in vivo with serum albumin, and with erythrocyte and lymphocyte membrane proteins (Bucala et al, 1984, 1982). Similar adduct formation by this process with the estrogen receptor could lead to inappropriate expression of hormonal action in estrogen target tissues and result in cell transformation and tissue specific carcinogenesis.

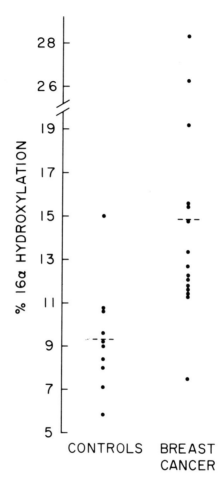

Figure 3. The reaction scheme between 16 α-hydroxyestrone (16α–OHE) and the ε-amino group of lysine residues, showing the adducts formed under nonreducing conditions by the Heyn's rearrangement and under reducing conditions with NaCNBH$_3$.

The results described above thus provide evidence that increase estrogen 16α-hydroxylase activity which is genetically encoded could constitute a marker for breast cancer risk and that the product of this enzyme 16α-hydroxyestrone could be an etiological factor in this disease.

Acknowledgment

This work was supported by grant CA22795 from the National Cancer Institute and grant HD19825 from the National Institute of Child Health and Human Development.

References

Beatson GT (1896). On the Treatment of Inoperable Cases of Carcinoma of the Mammary: Suggestions for a New Method with Illustrative Cases. Lancet 2:104-107.

Bradlow HL, Hersheopf RJ, Martucci CP, Fishman J. Estradiol 16α-Hydroxylation in the Mouse Correlates with Mammary Tumor Incidence and MMTV Presence. A Possible Model for the Hormonal Etiology of Breast Cancer in Man. Proc Natl Acad Sci (submitted)

Bucala R, Fishman J, Cerami A (1982). A Formation of Covalent Adducts between Cortisol and 16α-hydroxyestrone. A Possible Role in the Pathogenesis of Cortisol Toxicity and Systemic Lupus Erythematosis. Proc Natl Acad Sci USA 79:3320-3324.

Bucala R, Fishman J, Cerami A (1984). The Reaction of 16α-hydroxyestrone with Erythrocytes In Vivo and In Vitro. Eur J Biochem 140:593-598.

Bulbrook RD, Swain MC, Wang DY, Hayward JL, Kumaoka S, Tokatoni O, Abe O, Utsunomiya J. Breast Cancer in Britain and Japan: Plasma Estradiol, Estriol and Progesterone and their Urinary Metabolites in Normal British and Japanese Women. Eur J Cancer 12:725:735.

Clark JH, Paszko Z, Peck EJ Jr (1977). Nuclear Binding and Retention of the Receptor Estrogen Complex: Relation to the Agonistic and Antogonistic Properties of Estriol.

Endocrinology 100:91-96.

Cole P, Brown JB, MacMahon B (1976). Oestrogen Profiles of Parous and Nulliparous Women. Lancet 596-599.

Fishman J, Bradlow HL, Gallagher TF (1960). Oxidative Metabolism of Estradiol. J Biol Chem 235:3104-3107.

Fishman J, Schneider J, Anderson K, Kappas, A. (1980). Radiometric Analysis of Biological Oxidations in Man: Sex Differences in Estradiol Metabolism. Proc Natl Acad Sci USA 77:4957-4961.

Hellman L, Fishman J, Zumoff B, Cassouto J, Gallagher TF (1967). Studies of Estradiol Transformation in Women with Breast Cancer. J Clin Endocrinol Metab 27:1087-1092.

Hellman L, Zumoff B, Fishman J, Gallagher TF (1971). Peripheral Metabolism of ^{3}H-Estradiol and the Excretion of Endogenous Estrone and Estriol Glucosiduronate in Women with Breast Cancer. J Clin Endocrinol Metab 33:138-144.

Hilgar AG (1968). Uterotropic Evaluation of Steroids and Other Compounds. In: Uterotropic Biossay Data, editors AG Hilgar, LC French. National Cancer Institute, 58-70.

Huggins C, Jensen EV (1957). The Depression of Estrone Induced Uterine Growth by Phenolic Estrogens with Oxygenated Functions as Positions 6 or 16: The Impeded Estrogens. J Exp Med 102:335-346.

Korenman SG (1980). Oestrogen Window Hypothesis of the Actiology of Breast Cancer. Lancet, 700-703.

Lahita RG, Bradlow HL, Kunkel HG, Fishman J, (1979). Alterations of Estrogen Metabolism in Systemic Lupus Erythematosus. Arthritis and Rheumatism 22:1195-1198.

Lahita R, Bradlow HL, Kunkel HG, Fishman J, (1981). Increased 16 α-hydroxylation of Estradiol in Systemic Lupus Erythematosus. J Clin Endocrinol Metab 53:174-178.

Lemon HM, Wotiz HH, Parsons L, Mozdan PJ (1966) Reduced Estriol Excretion in Patients with Breast Cancer Prior to Endocrine Therapy. JAMA 196:112-120.

Lemon HM (1972). Genetic Predisposition of Carcinoma of the Breast: Multiple Human Genotypes for Estrogen 16α -hydroxylase Activity in Caucasians. J Surg Onc 4:255-273.

MacMahon B, Cole P, Lin TM, Lowe CR, Mirra AP (1970). Age at First Birth and Breast Cancer Risk. Bulletin WHO 33:209-221.

MacMahon B, Cole P, Brown JB (1973). Etiology of Human Breast Cancer: A Review. J Natl Cancer Inst 50:21-42.

MacMahon B, Cole P, Brown JB, Aoki K, Lin TM, Morgan RW, Woo NC (1974). Urine Oestrogen Profiles of Asian and North American Women. Int J Cancer 14:161-167.

MacMahon B, Trichopoulos D, Brown J, Anderson AP, Cole P, Dewaard F, Kauranicmi T (1982). Age of Menarche, Urine Estrogens and Breast Cancer Risk. Int J Cancer 30:427-431.

Martucci C, Fishman J (1977). Direction of Estradiol Metabolism as Control of its Hormonal Action: Uterotrophic Activity of Estradiol Metabolites. Endocrinolgy 101: 709-715.

Poortman J (1980). In: Reviews on Endocrine Related Cancer, No 6, editor B.L. Stoll.

Rudali G, Apiou F, Muel B (1975). Mammary Cancer Produced in Mice with Estriol. Eur J Cancer 4:39-41.

Schneider J, Kinne D, Fracchia A, Pierce V, Anderson KE, Bradlow HL, Fishman J (1982). J. Abnormal Oxidative Metabolism of Estradiol in Women with Breast Cancer. Proc Natl Acad Sci USA 79:3047-3051.

Trichopoulos D, MacMahon B, Cole P (1972). Menopause and Breast Cancer Risk. J Natl Cancer Inst 98:601-613.

Zumoff B, Fishman J, Cassouto J, Gallagher TF, Hellman L (1968). Influence on Age and Sex on Normal Estradiol Mmetabolism. J Clin Endocrinol Metab 28:937-941.

Zumoff B, Bradlow HL, Gallagher TF, Hellman L, (1971) Decreased Conversion of Androgens to Normal 17-ketosteroid Metabolites: A Nonspecific Consequence of illness. J Clin Endocrinol Metab 32:824-829.

Zumoff B, Fishman J, Bradlow HL, Hellman L,
   (1975). Hormone Profiles in Hormone-
   dependent Cancers. Cancer Res 35:3365-3369.

**Tumor Markers and Their Significance in the Management
of Breast Cancer, pages 105–123**
© **1986 Alan R. Liss, Inc.**

ESTROGEN REGULATION OF H59 ANTIGEN IN VIVO AND IN VITRO[1]

Fred J. Hendler, Kelly Patrick, Diane House

Department of Internal Medicine
The University of Texas Health Science Center
Dallas, Texas   75235

ABSTRACT

H59 antibody, a murine monoclonal antibody, recognizes
a cell surface peptide of approximately 30,000 MW which is
estrogen regulated. The data supporting this conclusion
have been generated from in vitro systems and indirectly
from human tissue specimens. The antigen is detected only
in estrogen regulated breast cancer cells in culture and is
not detected in two estrogen independent cell lines, R_3 and
R_{27}, which were derived from estrogen sensitive MCF-7 that
contain the antigen. The antigen is increased in estrogen
stimulated cells and decreased in tamoxifen inhibited
cells. H59 antigen appears estrogen regulated in human
breast colostrum and milk and in endometrium. The antigen
is found in 40% of breast cancer and most, if not all,
normal breast tissue. In the more than 300 breast cancer
specimens studied, H59 antigen was detected in predominate-
ly estrogen and/or progesterone receptor containing tumors.
This antigen was found only in about 50% of ER positve
tumors. When the presence of H59 was compared to other
prognostic factors in breast cancer, it appeared to be an
independent variable and correlated only with the presence
of estrogen and progesterone receptor. The antigen can be
detected in normal serum, and studies are underway to determine if it will serve as a circulating marker protein in
hormone dependent breast cancer.

INTRODUCTION

H59 antibody (H59 Ab) was synthesized as part of an effort to develop an antibody to an estrogen regulated cell surface antigen (1-4). The rationale for this approach was to identify such a protein which might be a more useful marker of in vivo estrogen responsiveness than the presence of estrogen (ER) and progesterone receptor (PR). Only a few estrogen regulated proteins in breast cancer have been identified and their utility as markers of in vivo estrogen responsiveness have not been established (5-12).

Rather than isolating an estrogen regulated cellular protein, ZR-75-1 cells, an estrogen sensitive human breast cancer tissue culture cell line, were used as the immunogen and mouse-mouse hybridomas were produced. The initial screen segregated hybridomas which reacted only with estrogen sensitive cell lines from those that did not. H59 Ab was selected on this basis and subsequently shown to have minimal binding to non-breast cancer cells (1-4). The antibody has been shown to detect the H59 antigen (H59 Ag) in approximately 40% of breast cancers and most, if not all, normal and hyperplastic breast epithelia (4). Of the more than 300 breast tumors studied, those which contain the antigen have either ER and/or PR. However, only slightly more than 50% of the ER and PR positive tumors contain the antigen (4).

The H59 Ag has been partially purified and characterized in breast cancer cells and normal human tissues. In its dissociated form it has a molecular weight of approximately 30,000; this does not react with H59 Ab (12). In cell lysates H59 Ag is greater than 200,000 daltons. It appears to be estrogen regulated in vivo and in vitro and can be detected in human sera. Thus, it may be an excellent marker for estrogen sensitive breast cancer.

MATERIALS AND METHODS

Monoclonal Antibodies

H59, H71, and H72 IgM antibodies were isolated from hybridoma cultures obtained from the fusion of ZR-75-1 immunized BALB/c spleen cells and mouse myeloma cells (1-4). The antigen to which the antibodies were binding was characterized by a direct and indirect radioimmunoassay against a panel of glutaraldehyde fixed normal and cancer cells and acetone fixed cryosections obtained from normal tissues and human tumors. Antibodies were radiolabeled with [^{125}I]-iodine using lactoperoxidase to a specific activity of 2 to 10,000 trichloracetic acid (TCA) precipitable cpm per ng of antibody protein.

Tissue Specimens

Normal and breast cancer specimens were obtained from patients undergoing biopsies for diagnostic purposes at Baylor University Medical Center, Parkland Memorial Hospital, and St. Paul's Medical Center (Dallas, TX). Colostrum and breast milk were obtained from pregnant and lactating women with informed consent. Endometrium and serum were obtained with informed consent from women undergoing hysterectomy at Parkland Memorial Hospital.

Tissue Radioimmunoassay

The direct tissue radioimmunoassay which we have used extensively is well described (1-4,14-16). Cryosections were fixed with 50% acetone-phosphate buffered saline (PBS) and subsequently reacted with radiolabeled antibody (2×10^5 cpm in 100 ul PBS containing 50% calf serum) for 3 hrs at 25°C. Following extensive washing of the tissue sections, X-ray film was placed over the sections and exposed for 16 hrs. Binding was observed by at least two observers independently and scored on a scale of 0-4+ by either scanning densitometry or observation (4,14,15). Three plus or greater binding over infiltrating tumor was scored as a positive result.

Cell Culture

Either ZR-75-1 or MCF-7 cells were maintained in Richter's improved minimal essential media containing 10% charcoal treated calf serum and 10^{-7}M insulin. At a density of slightly less than 50% confluence, the media was changed to serum free plus insulin and 24 hrs later either estradiol (10^{-8}M), tamoxifen (10^{-7}M), estradiol plus tamoxifen, or no hormones were added to the cultures. One set of cultured cells received [^{35}S]-methionine (10 uCi/ml) 31 hours after the addition of hormones. A duplicate set of cultures received no radioactivity. At 36 hrs cells were harvested by scraping and separated from the media by centrifugation. Cells were lysed with 1% nonidet P-40 (NP-40) in phosphate buffered saline (PBS) and a 1×10^5G supernatant cytosol prepared. For studies quantitating the antigen present, the lysate was chromatographed in 1% NP-40 PBS on Sephacryl 300 and the high molecular weight (HMW) fraction, tubes 13-17, were pooled (Figure 2).

Antigen Quantitation

To measure the antigen present in cell lysate, media, and human breast milk and endometrium, a quantitative "immunoblot" radioimmunoassay was used (17). Unlabeled antibody or antigen containing material was bound to nitrocellulose filter paper (0.45 u, S&S, Keene, NH) which had been placed in a slotted apparatus (S&S). The filter paper was air dried and additional binding sites were blocked by incubation in PBS containing 3% bovine serum albumin and 1% NP-40. The filter papers were reacted with the appropriate [^{125}I]-labeled antibody at 37°C for 16 hrs and washed with 4 changes of 1% NP-40 PBS with 10% calf serum at 37°C. The filters were exposed to X-ray film (XAR, Kodak, Rochester, NY) in cassettes with Cronex enhancers (Dupont, Wilmington, DE) at -70°C. Up to 10 ug of protein can be quantitatively bound to the nitrocellulose filter paper using the slot blotter. The amount of antigen or antibody bound was quantitated by scanning densitometry (E-C Apparatus, St. Petersburg, FL) of an autoradiograph.

Serum Assay

The level of H59 Ag in human serum was determined using the quantitative "immunoblot" technique described above. However, in order to detect the level of antigen in serum required collection of the HMW fraction from serum which had been passed over a Sephacryl 300 column (Figure 2). 10 ug of this pooled fraction was bound to nitrocellulose and the amount of antigen detected quantitated by comparison with ZR-75 cell lysate treated similarly.

RESULTS AND DISCUSSION

The Relationship of H59 Ag to Estrogen Receptor in Breast Cancer Specimens

H59 Ab and two other antibodies, H71 Ab and H72 Ab, which bind to normal and malignant breast cancer cells have been reacted with 332 cryopreserved tissue sections from breast cancer biopsy (259 from primary tumors) and 111 sections from benign breast disease. H59 recognizes antigens which are present only in breast, ovarian, and prostate cancers; whereas, H71 and H72 antibodies recognize differentiation antigens which are present in breast and other tissues (Table 1). Using these three antibodies, approximately 85% of tumor specimens are bound (4); the addition of H88 (18), a fourth antibody with similar specificity increased the binding by antibodies to approximately 90% of tumor specimens (19). The binding of the antibodies to the first 152 specimens has been correlated with the ER and PR content of the tumor tissue (4). Almost all of the specimens which bound H59 Ab contained significant levels of ER and/or PR. H71 Ab and H72 Ab bound specimens regardless of the steroid receptor content. Hence, H59 Ag is associated with the presence of receptors in breast cancers. The data suggest that it is not a constituitive protein in receptor negative tissue as has been observed with the 52K protein (5,6). The tight correlation between the presence of ER and H59 Ag implies that the antigen is estrogen regulated in breast cancers.

TABLE 1: Monoclonal Antibody to Adenocarcinoma Biopsy
Specimens

Cryopreserved tissue sections from primary adenocarcinomas
were reacted with three monoclonal antibodies derived from
breast cancer cells with an irrelevant control antibody,
MTS, and evaluated according to the Methods.

Tissue	Number of Specimens	Antibody (Specimens Bound)		
		H59	H71	H72
Breast	259	103	126	170
Other Adenocarcinomas				
Lung	20	0	16	11
Ovary	5	3	2	4
Prostate	5	2	1	0
Pancreas	5	0	2	2
Colon	5	0	3	2
Stomach	5	0	2	2
Renal	5	0	0	1

Since H59 Ab binding was associated with the presence
of steroid hormone receptors, it might be an important
prognostic factor in breast cancer. To determine if it is
an independent variable, antibody binding was compared with
other prognostic indicators. There was no apparent relationship of H59 binding with tumor size, the presence of
involved axillary lymph nodes, the stage of the tumor, the
age of the patient, or nuclear grade (19). However, the
binding of H59 and at least either H71 or H72 was associated with a higher ER or PR level (4). Similarly, in this
patient population, the presence of ER and/or PR appears to
be independent of these other prognostic factors. In 73
biopsy specimens of metastatic disease, the binding of H59
was significantly less than the percentage of those patients where primary disease was evaluated (20 vs 37.5%) (p
<0.01), and those specimens binding no antibody increased
to 25% of the population studied (19). Thus, H59 and other
antibody binding may be important prognostic factors and
independent of other variables. It will be necessary to
follow these patients, establishing the time of disease

recurrence and survival. Another approach which can be
done with these antibodies since they bind paraffin embedded tissue is to evaluate patients retrospectively in the
disease free interval when survival and response to therapy
have been determined.

The Estrogen Regulation of H59 Ag in Cultured Breast Cancer
Cells

At least eight peptides are produced in a continuous
cultured breast cancer cell lines as a response to estradiol (5-12). As yet, none of these proteins have been
associated with steroid responsive breast cancer in vivo.
These proteins appear to be constituitive in ER negative
cell lines and in estrogen resistant cell lines with ER and
PR. Therefore, it may be difficult to demonstrate that the
presence of these proteins in a tumor or serum is a useful
marker of hormone dependent breast cancer.

H59 binds to either one or possibly two peptides of
approximately 30K daltons. This antigen is localized to
the cell surface of most breast cancer and normal breast
duct cells and appears to be secreted by cultured tumor
cells, normal duct cells, and many breast tumors (1-4). It
is not constituitive in the cell lines studied which either
lack ER or those that have ER and PR but are no longer
estrogen regulated (3,4).

To determine whether H59 Ag is estrogen regulated in
human breast cancer, the H59, H71, and H72 antigen levels
have been measured in two cell lines which are model systems of estrogen regulation in vitro, ZR-75-1 and MCF-7
cells (13,19). Estrogen stimulation was demonstrated by
incubating ZR-75-1 and MCF-7 cells with estrogen, inhibiting cells with tamoxifen, and reversing the tamoxifen effects with estrogen. Total incorporation of ^{35}S-methionine
into ZR-75-1 and MCF-7 TCA precipitable material in cell
lysates were stimulated 35% and 100% by 10^{-8}M estradiol,
respectively; tamoxifen inhibited incorporation into both
ZR-75-1 and MCF-7 lysates 30% and 20%, respectively. Estrogen was able to overcome the effects of tamoxifen in
both cell lines. Estrogen stimulated the incorporation of
^{35}S-methionine into H59 antigen 4.5 and 3.5-fold in ZR-75-1
and MCF-7 cell lysates. The tamoxifen effectively dimin-

ished ^{35}S-methionine incorporation into H59 antigen in ZR-75-1 and MCF-7 lysates by 80% and 35%, respectively. The addition of estradiol to cells containing tamoxifen overcame the effect of tamoxifen, an H59 antigen, in both cell lines.

The Expression of H59 Ag in Normal Human Tissues and Secretions

1. <u>Antigen content in colostrum and milk.</u> The responsiveness to estrogens in breast tissue represents a retained differentiated function of normal breast glandular tissue. If H59 Ag were estrogen regulated in normal breast, the antigen level in breast milk should vary with the circulating level of estrogens. The two major milk proteins, casein and alpha-lactalbumin, are synthesized in approximately 20% of breast cancers (20,21). Both of these proteins are regulated by prolactin, and there is no correlation between these proteins and either the presence of estrogen receptor or the response to a sex steroid hormone manipulation (22,23).

H59, H71, and H72 antigens have been measured in human breast milk from 7 women obtained prior to delivery and for up to 1 and 1/2 years postpartum (18). Since H71 is clearly hormone independent, its level served as control for the change in protein content with lactation and the synthesis of casein and alpha-lactalbumin. H59 Ag was present in the colostrum and breast milk of all specimens that have been studied. H59 Ag was highest in colostrum and immediately postpartum (24 hrs) with respect to H71. It steadily began to decrease after 24 hrs postpartum, reaching its nadir at the first week and remaining essentially constant until menstruation began again. H72 Ag decreased similarly to H59 with lactation. Breast duct cells are regulated by estrogen and progesterone until parturition, and following parturition regulation is via progesterone and prolactin. Thus, the decrease in H59 Ag was consistent with these being under estrogen regulation in normal breast cells.

2. <u>Antigen content in normal endometrium.</u> Since H59 can be detected in normal endometrium and oviduct as well as 50% of endometrial and ovarian cancer (Table 1), another approach to demonstrate estrogen regulation has been to

measure the H59 antigen content of endometrial tissue.
Using the immunoblot technique H59, H71, and H72 antigens
have been detected in endometrium. The level of antigen is
comparable to that detected in ZR-75-1 cells where the
antigen represents from 1×10^{-3} to 1×10^{-4} of the cell lysate
protein. The amount of antigens present have been corre-
lated with the endometrial phase from 13 specimens obtained
at hysterectomy (Figure 1). H59 Ag and H72 significantly
fluctuate with the menstrual cycle; whereas, H71 Ag, which
is not affected by estrogen, does not. This variation in
the antigen content is presumably secondary to circulating
estrogen level. Thus, this association further supports
the thesis that H59 Ag is estrogen regulated in vivo.

    3. Antigen content in normal serum. Initially, we
were unable to detect the presence of H59, H71, and H72
antigens in sera from patients. In purifying the antigens
from ZR-75-1 and MCF-7 cell lysates, the antigens were
localized to the HMW fraction (<150,000) using column chromatography (Figure 2). The HMW chromatographic fraction
gave an 8-fold concentration of the antigens from ZR-75-1
cell lysates. Since this fraction represents 4% of the
serum proteins, the theoretic concentration of the antigen
in the HMW serum fraction was 25-fold. With the immunoblot
assay, a 1/20,000 dilution of antigen can be detected in
serum (Figure 3). Sera from four patients on whom endometrial tissue has been obtained were chromatographed and
reacted with the three antibodies in the immunoblot assay
(Figure 4). Using the ZR-75-1 HMW fraction dilutions as
standards (Figure 5), the amount of antigens in serum from
4 patients from whom endometrial tissue was obtained was
determined (Figure 6). The level is approximately 1/2000
of the antigen concentration observed in ZR-75-1 lysates
and endometrium homogenates. We have begun to use this
assay to determine the level of antigen in serum from additional normal patients and patients with breast cancer.

FIGURE 1.   Binding of monoclonal antibodies to endometrium.
Uterus was obtained from patients undergoing hysterectomies
for dysfunctional uterine bleeding secondary to myofibro-
mata.   The normal endometrium was removed by scraping and
homogenized in PBS in 1% NP-40.   Following centrifugation a
100,000 G supernatant was obtained.   10 ug of this supernatant was bound to nitrocellulose and reacted with 1×10^6
TCA precipitable cpm of radiolabeled monoclonal antibody
according to the immunoblot technique. The amount of antibody binding was determined from X-ray film exposed for 16
hrs. The density was subsequently determined by scanning
densitometry.   The endometrial phase of the tissue was
determined morphologically.   The antibodies reacted were
H59 □, H71+, H72 ◊ .

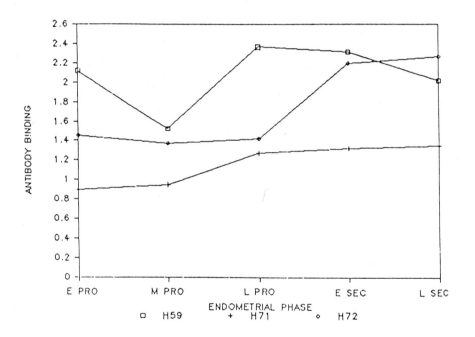

FIGURE 2

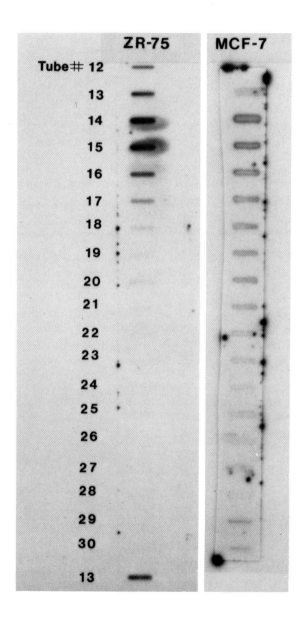

(Figure legend on next page)

FIGURE 2. Column chromatography of H59 Ag in cell lysates. ZR-75-1 or MCF-7 breast cancer cells were grown in the presence of Richter's improved minimum essential media with supplementation of insulin (10^{-7}M), estradiol (10^{-8}M), and 10% calf serum. The cells were collected by scraping at 75% confluence, washed and lysed with 1% NP-40 in PBS. The 100,000 G cell lysate supernatant (1 ml) was subjected to Sephacryl 300 column chromatograpy (column dimensions 1x40 cm) and 1 ml fractions were collected. 1 ug of protein for each fraction was bound to nitrocellulose and reacted with 1×10^6 cpm [^{125}I]-H59 antibody according to the immunoblot techniques. The filters were washed and exposed to X-ray film for either 16 hrs at -70°C (ZR-75-1) or 72 hrs (MCF-7) and developed. The fraction numbers are listed on the left and the cell lines above. There are two fraction numbers 13 for ZR-75 since the complete sample was too great a volume for a single slot. Fractions 12-16 were pooled to form the HMW fraction in subsequent experiments.

FIGURE 3. The binding of ZR-75 cell lysate to nitrocellulose.
A 100,000 G ZR-75-1 cell lysate was chromatographed on Sephacryl 300. The HMW fractions were pooled and the protein determined. From that sample a range of concentration from 0.005 ug to 10 ug were bound to nitrocellulose in an admixture with from 10 ug to 0 ug of HMW calf serum which had been similarly chromatographed; thus, the amount of protein added to the nitrocellulose was constant. The filter was reacted with either 1×10^6 cpm of H59 Ab or a nonspecific antibody of the same isotype (MTS). The filters were washed, exposed for 72 hrs at -70°C and developed.

FIGURE 3

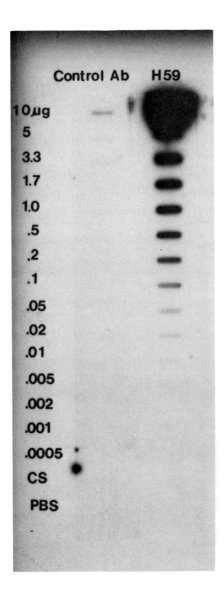

FIGURE 4. Detection of monoclonal antibody binding in human serum.
Blood was collected from 4 patients who were about to undergo a hysterectomy. The HMW fraction of sera was obtained by Sephacryl 300 chromatography (Figure 2) and 10 ug of protein was bound to nitrocellulose. 1 ug of the HMW fraction from an endometrial specimen was similarly bound to the filter. The nitrocellulose filters were reacted with 1×10^6 cpm of radiolabeled H59, H71, and H72 antibodies and washed with standard immunoblot techniques. The X-ray film was exposed for 72 hrs at -70°C. The dilution study of ZR-75-1 lysate HMW fraction was reacted, exposed, and developed simultaneously (Figure 3).

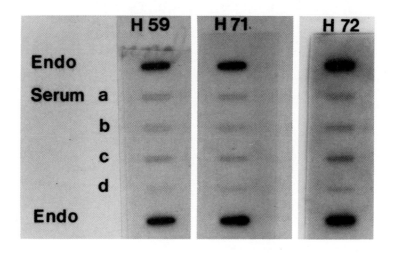

FIGURE 5. Scanning densitometry of HMW ZR-75-1 cell lysate
dilutions.
The autoradiograph in Figure 3 was scanned with a recording
densitometer (E-C, St. Petersburg, FL). The intensity of
H59 Ab binding was plotted according to the amount of HMW
fraction ZR-75-1 cell lysate which was bound to nitrocellulose. The curve generated in a straight line with a coef-
ficient of regression of 0.986.

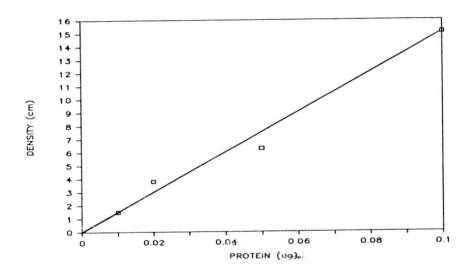

FIGURE 6. Quantitation of monoclonal antibody binding to
human sera.
The HMW fractions of ZR-75-1 and sera (Figures 3,4) had
been reacted with radiolabeled antibody simultaneously, the
filters washed, exposed to X-ray film for 72 hrs at -70°C,
and developed together. The autoradiographs were scanned
with a densitometer and the intensity of antibody binding
calculated (Figure 5). The binding of sera was related to
the intensity of antibody binding to HMW ZR-75-1 cell lysate. The antibodies bound were H59□, H71+, and H72◊. The
control Ab, MTS, demonstrated no detectable binding above
filter paper controls.

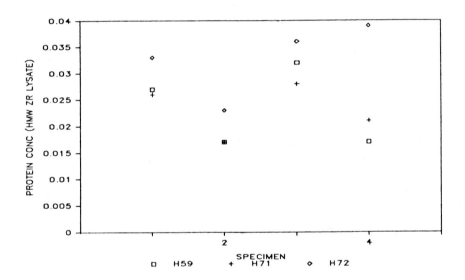

CONCLUSIONS

The H59 antigen has been detected only in other normal tissues and tumors which are known to be sex steroid hormone regulated. The H59 antigen has been associated with the presence of ER in tumor tissue and is estrogen regulated in vitro. It has been detected in metastatic tissue and both benign and malignant axillary nodes. It is present in normal sera. Thus, H59 antigen has the potential for being an excellent marker for estrogen regulated breast cancer. However, the following must be demonstrated to establish the antigen's utility: 1) the binding of the antibody to tumor is associated with tumors that respond to sex steroid manipulations, 2) the H59 Ag can be detected with some degree of selectivity in serum from patients with disseminated breast cancer, and 3) H59 Ag fluctuates with the tumor burden and response to a therapeutic manipulation.

REFERENCES

1. Hendler et al (1981). Characterization of a monoclonal antibody to human breast cancer cells. Trans Assoc Amer Phys 94: 217-224.
2. Yuan et al (1982). Characterization of a monoclonal antibody reactive with a subset of human breast tumors. J Natl Cancer Inst 68: 719-728.
3. Hendler FJ, Yuan D (1983). Binding of H59 and other monoclonal antibodies to human breast cancer. In Chabner BA (ed): "Rational Basis for Chemotherapy," New York: Alan R. Liss, pp 309-314.
4. Hendler FJ, Yuan D (1985). The relationship of monoclonal antibody binding to estrogen and progesterone receptor content in breast cancer. Cancer Res 45: 421-429.
5. Westley B, Rochefort H (1980). A secreted glycoprotein induced by estrogen in human breast cancer cell lines. Cell 20: 353-362.
6. Vignon et al (1984). Induction of two estrogen-responsive proteins by antiestrogens in R_{27}, a tamoxifen-resistant clone of MCF_7 cells. Cancer Res 44: 2084-2088.

7. Westley B, Rochefort H (1979). Estradiol induced proteins in the MCF$_7$ human breast cancer cell line. Biochem Biophys Res Commun 90: 410-416.
8. Edwards et al (1980). Estrogen induced synthesis of specific proteins in human breast cancer cells. Biochem Biophys Res Commun 93: 804-812.
9. Mairesse et al (1980). Estrogen-induced protein in the human breast cancer cell line MCF$_7$. Biochem Biophys Res Commun 97: 1251-1257.
10. Huff KK, Lippman ME (1984). Hormonal control of plasminogen activator secretion in ZR-75-1 human breast cancer cells in culture. Endocrinology 114: 1702-1701.
11. Massot et al (1984). The estrogen-regulated 52 K protein and plasminogen activators released by MCF$_7$ cells are different. Mol Cell Endocrinol 35: 167-175.
12. Chalbos D, Rochefort H (1984). A 250-kilodalton cellular protein is induced by progestins in two human breast cancer cell lines MCF$_7$ and T$_{47}$D. Biochem Biophys Res Commun 121: 421-427.
13. Hendler FJ (1984). H59 antigen is estrogen regulated in breast cancer cells. Breast Cancer Res Treat 4: 337.
14. Cowley et al (1984). The amount of EGF receptor is elevated on squamous cell carcinomas. Cancer Cells 1: 5-10.
15. Hendler FJ, Ozanne BW (1984). Squamous cell cancers express increased EGF receptors. J Clin Invest 74: 647-651.
16. Hendler FJ, House D (1985). The presence of breast cancer antigens in uninvolved axillary lymph nodes. Cancer Res (accepted for publication).
17. Towbin et al (1979). Electrophoretic transfer of proteins from polyacrylamide gels to nitrocellulose sheets: procedures and some applications. Proc Natl Acad Sci USA 76: 4350-4354.
18. Hendler et al (1985). Identification of two tumors coexistent at three separate sites using monoclonal antibodies. Submitted for publication.
19. Hendler et al (1985). Clinical studies on cell surface estrogen-regulated proteins. In Ceriani RL (ed): "Proceedings of the International Workshop on Monoclonal Antibodies and Breast Cancer," Boston: Martinus Nijhoff Publishing, in press.

20. Monaco et al (1977). Casein production by human breast cancer. Cancer Res 37: 749-754.
21. Kleinberg DL (1975). Human alpha-lactalbumin: measurement in serum and in breast cancer organ cultures by radioimmunoassay. Science 190: 276-278.
22. Monaco ME, Lippman ME. Unpublished data.
23. Hall et al (1981). Alpha-lactalbumin is not a marker of human hormone-dependent breast cancer. Nature 290: 602-604.

Tumor Markers and Their Significance in the Management of Breast Cancer, pages 125–140
© 1986 Alan R. Liss, Inc.

THE 52 K PROTEIN : AN ESTROGEN REGULATED MARKER OF CELL PROLIFERATION IN HUMAN MAMMARY CELLS

H. Rochefort, F. Capony, M. Garcia, M. Morisset, I. Touïtou and F. Vignon

Unité d'Endocrinologie Cellulaire et Moléculaire (U148) I.N.S.E.R.M.
60, rue de Navacelles - 34100 Montpellier France

1. INTRODUCTION

Estrogens promote the genesis and growth of human breast cancers by an unknown mechanism (1). In this paper, we illustrate how some estrogen-regulated proteins may serve both as potential markers in the management of breast cancer and as intermediate steps to understand the control of cell proliferation by estrogens. The aim of our study was two-fold : the first was to search better marker(s) for hormone responsiveness than the ones currently available. The assay of estrogen and progesterone receptors is useful (2), but there are many examples of discrepancies between the regulation by estrogen and antiestrogens of the progesterone receptor and of cell proliferation. Hence, other estrogen-regulated proteins more closely related to the hormonal regulation of tumor growth would be usefull. Our second objective was to improve our understanding of the mechanism by which estrogen stimulates the growth of hormone-responsive breast cancer. This could provide the means of interfering with estrogen-induced tumor proliferation using neutralizing antibodies. To reach these objectives, human metastatic breast cancer cell lines (MCF7, T47D, ZR75-1...) are excellent systems. They contain estrogen receptors, progesterone receptors, glucocorticoid and androgen receptors and their growth is stimulated by estrogens (3)(4)(5) and inhibited by progestins (6) and synthetic antiestrogens (3). These cells (mostly MCF7 cells) have been used by several laboratories to detect new estrogen-regulated markers and to study the mechanism of growth stimulation by estrogens.

In this respect, the estrogen-regulated proteins secreted by hormone-responsive cells are particularly attractive for several reasons :

First, these proteins can be released into the blood, and serve as potential circulating markers of hormone dependency in breast cancer.

Second, some of these proteins or peptides released into the extracellular medium can totally modulate the growth of the producing cells (autocrine) (7), or neighboring cells (paracrine). Therefore, they may serve as second messengers of steroid hormones for regulating the nonspecific mitogenic response.

Third, these proteins are relatively easy to detect and assay, contrary to cellular proteins (8).

For the past 5 years, we have been extensively studying proteins which are specifically regulated by estrogens in MCF7 cells and which are secreted by the cells into the culture medium (8).

Major contributions in the field are cited in recent reviews on the estrogen-induced proteins in breast cancer cell lines (9)(10)(11).

In this report, we mostly describe results from our laboratory concerning: 1. The general methodology for studying hormone-regulated proteins secreted by cell lines, and the general properties of the 52 K protein in MCF7 cells. 2. The development and use of monoclonal antibodies to the 52 K protein, showing its potential as a tissue marker in breast cancer. 3. The relationship between different estrogen-regulated secretory proteins and the control of cell proliferation, with recent evidence for a mitogenic activity of the 52 K protein.

2. EVIDENCE FOR ESTROGEN-REGULATED PROTEINS SECRETED BY MCF7 CELLS AND PROPERTIES OF THE 52 K PROTEIN

A general method for detecting steroid-regulated proteins involves labeling of the proteins in cell culture with ^{35}S-methionine and analyzing them according to their molecular weight after dissociation using SDS-poly-acrylamide gel electrophoresis followed by fluorography of the gel and scanning of the different bands (Fig. 1). This approach generally requires 2D gel analysis (12) in order to discriminate the induced cellular proteins. However, analysis of proteins released into the medium is easier, since their pattern is generally simpler and can therefore be carried out using one-dimensional gel analysis. The

Figure 1. General procedure for demonstrating sex steroid regulated proteins

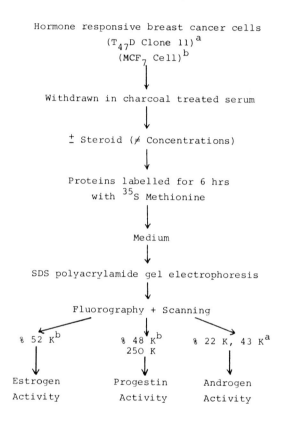

Detailed methodology for cell culture, hormone treatment, labeling and analysis of proteins are reported elsewhere (4)(6)(8).

a. T47D cells (clone 11) were provided by Dr I Keydar (Tel-Aviv University, Israel). T47D cells are also available at the Mason Research Institute (1530 East Jefferson Street, Rockville, Maryland 29852).

b. MCF7 cells were provided by the Michigan Cancer Foundation and Marc Lippman and are used to define estrogen activity (10).

major difficulty is to remove all the estrogens from the
serum and media used in the control (non estrogen-treated)
sample (13).

Using this technique, sex-steroid-regulated proteins
have been detected and defined according to their molecular
weight. Progestin and androgen-regulated proteins have
recently been described in T47D cells and will not be
considered here (14). In MCF7 cells, estrogens increase the
production of most secreted proteins and more specifically
that of two proteins of 52,000 and 160,000 daltons (8). The
52 K protein has been characterized over the past 5 years.
It is a glycoprotein, N-glycosylated with high mannose
oligosaccharide chains (15). The stimulation of production
in the medium is seen as early as 12 hours after the
beginning of estradiol treatment and is restricted to
hormones which can bind to and activate the estrogen
receptor present in the cells (10). There is a good
correlation between the in vitro binding affinity of
hormones to the estrogen receptor and the biological
activity of the 52 K protein, as defined in
dose-response-curve experiments on MCF7 cells (DE50).
Nonsteroidal antiestrogens (Tamoxifen and 4-hydroxy-
tamoxifen) alone have no effect on this protein but can
inhibit its production under estrogen stimulation. However,
the 52 K protein is not a general marker for the action of
mitogens, since it is not stimulated by prolactin, insulin,
or epidermal growth factor (Vignon et al., unpublished)
which stimulate the growth of MCF7 cells. Another protein
(160 K) which is not retained by Concanavalin A-Sepharose,
has not been purified and characterized. Since the 52 K
protein is produced in small amounts by estrogen-treated
MCF7 cells (15 ng/ml of medium), accounting for 20 to 40 %
of all the labeled proteins released into the culture
medium, we purified it in two steps. The 52 K protein was
first, partially purified on Con A-Sepharose from 25 l of
medium conditioned by MCF7 cells. In collaboration with
CLIN-MIDY/SANOFI Research Laboratory (Dr B. Pau), monoclonal antibodies (MAbs) were raised, cloned and purified
after fusion of mice lymphocytes with the murine myeloma
P3-X63-Ag8-653 (16). The secreted protein was then purified
to homogeneity using an immunoaffinity column (17) and
characterized as a single peptide which is both
glycosylated (high mannose chains) and phosphorylated (18).
In the cell extract, 3 species of 52,000, 48,000 and 34,000
daltons are recovered. The two lower molecular weight
proteins are more abundant and result from the processing

of the 52,000 protein, as shown by pulse chase experiments
(17). The structure and function of the purified secreted
protein are now being studied.

3. USE OF MONOCLONAL ANTIBODIES TO DETECT AND ASSAY THE 52 K PROTEIN IN DIFFERENT TISSUES

The 7 MAbs that were cloned and purified, are all of
the IgG1 isotype and their KDs range from 0.35 to 2.3 nM
(Table 1). The antibodies specifically recognize a secreted
and a cellular 52 K protein as evidenced by double
immunoprecipitation and by immunoblotting after electrophoretic separation and transfer. These antibodies have
been used both to assay the 52 K protein in soluble samples
and to detect it in cell or tissue sections (19).

Table 1. Characterization of the monoclonal antibodies to the Mr 52,000 protein

		Subclass	Affinity (KD) in nM	Specificity for Mr 52,000 protein	
				double immuno	immunoblot
	M1G8	IgG1	0.43	+	+
	M1H11	IgG1	2.86	+	+
Site 1	M6H10	IgG1	1.43	+	+
	D8F5	IgG1	1.25	+	+
	D11E2	IgG1	1.00	+	+
Site 2	D7E3	IgG1	0.83	+	+
Site 3	M4A3	IgG1	0.58	+	+

The 7 high-affinity antibodies can be classified into
three "sites" from their competition in double determinant
immunoradiometric assays. The D7E3 antibody (site 2) can be
used in a double determinant IRMA with any of the 5 "site
1" antibodies. Double immunoprecipitation and "western"
immunoblotting after electrophoretic transfer showed that
these antibodies exclusively recognize the 52 K protein in
culture medium.
(Modified from Ref 16 with the permission of the Editor).

A. Assay of the protein by double determinant IRMA

Double determinant immunoradiometric assay indicated that the 7 MAbs recognize at least three distinct regions of the Mr 52,000 protein and allow the 52 K protein to be assayed in biological fluids. With this sandwich assay, the concentration of the 52 K protein is determined by reference to a pure 52 K protein fraction assayed by silver staining. Our first results indicate that the MCF7 cells progressively accumulate the protein in the medium as a function of time (16). Other cell lines have recently been assayed for their ability to produce the 52 K protein. Non-human cells (rat...) and the estrogen-receptor-negative cell line HBL100 were non-productive (Table 2).

Table 2. Distribution of the 52 K protein in different human mammary cell lines and comparison to other estrogen-regulated parameters

	MARKERS OF RESPONSES TO ESTROGEN IN HUMAN CELL LINES						
	MCF_7	R_{27}	ZR_{75-1}	$T_{47}D$ $Cl.11$	BT_{20}	MDA MB_{231}	HBL_{100}
R_E	+	+	+	+	-	-	-
R_P	+	+	+	++	-	-	-
52 K PROTEIN	++	++	++	+	+	+	-
E_2 ON CELL PROLIFERATION	+	+	+	+	-	-	-

RE= estrogen receptor. RP= progesterone receptor. The 4 receptor-positive cell lines responded to estradiol both by producing the 52 K protein and by increasing their growth. The receptor-negative cell lines produced the 52 K protein constitutively at the same level whether estradiol was present or not. HBL100 derived from human milk epithelial cells produced no detectable 52 K protein in the culture medium. The concentration of the 52 K protein in the medium measured by double determinant IRMA (16) varied between 0,5 to 5 ng per µg DNA per day (+) and 5 to 20 ng per µg DNA per day (++).
(From Ref 10, 29 and Garcia & Derocq, unpublished).

All estrogen-receptor-positive cell lines tested produce the protein, but to a varying degree. For instance, T47D clone 11 cells have high concentrations of RP but produce low concentration of 52 K protein. In this cell line, other E_2- regulated proteins (60 kDa) are more abundant. Particularly interesting are the two estrogen-receptor-negative cell lines (BT20, MDA MB231) in which the 52 K protein is produced constitutively with or without estrogen.

B. Immunoperoxidase staining

These antibodies did not react with the external plasma membrane of MCF7 cells, as shown by immuno-fluorescence cell sorter analysis. By contrast, the cytoplasm of MCF7 cells was stained by the peroxidase antiperoxidase complex after plasma membrane permeation, suggesting that the protein is secreted by exocytosis rather than shedded from plasma membrane (16).

Using these monoclonal antibodies, we have examined frozen sections of several human tissues with the peroxidase-anti-peroxidase technique (19). Negative controls were routinely performed with an excess of antigen, or with irrelevant IgG antibodies showing the staining specificity. In 75 % of the primary breast cancers studied, specific staining was observed in the cytoplasm of epithelial cancer cells but not in the stroma. The samples that were not stained generally contained no detectable estrogen receptor. No staining was observed in 8 "normal" human mammary glands collected during reduction mammoplasties and in 9 "normal" uteri, regardless of whether tissues were collected in the follicular or luteal phase. Three endometrial cancers were also negative. Several normal human tissues have been examined. None, except sweat glands, have been shown to react with the antibodies to the 52 K protein. Although normal resting mammary glands were negative, benign mastopathies were frequently positive. The staining occurred mostly in the cytoplasm of ductal epithelial cells, and in the lumen of the cysts. A study on a hundred mastopathies with a comparison of adjacent sections for pathology diagnosis is in progress, in collaboration with the pathologists (Pr Pages) and clinicians (Pr Pujol) of Montpellier University. The first results on a limited number of samples suggest a more frequent positive reactivity in mastopathies with high risk of breast cancer (fibrocystic disease with hyperplasia, ductal hyperplasia) than in mastopathies without high risk (gynecomastia, adenosis, fibrous mastopathies...).

The tentative conclusions from these first results are the following :

a. The 52 K protein is a human specific marker. There was no reactivity with C3H mouse or DMBA or NMU rat mammary tumors (M. Garcia and A. Manni, unpublished).

b. The 52 K protein is not a general marker of estrogen responsiveness, unlike the progesterone receptor or the 24 K protein (11), since it is not found in endometrium.

c. The 52 K protein is specific for mammary tissue (and sweat glands) suggesting a relationship with apocrine glands.

d. The 52 K protein is a tumor and/or proliferation-associated marker. It was not detected in normal resting epithelial mammary cells (19) or in the culture medium after ^{35}S-methionine labeling (20). However, its presence at low concentrations has not been excluded. Its detection and quantification in fibrocystic disease appears to be a promising approach, since the protein may be useful in the diagnosis of breast cancer at early stages, and in helping to define high-risk mastopathies.

e. As a hormone-dependent marker of breast cancer, the 52 K protein is clearly estrogen-regulated in RE positive tumors. However, it can be produced constitutively in RE negative tumors. We are now collaborating with several cancer centers to correlate receptor assays and 52 K-protein detection in breast cancer. These studies have to be completed before the clinical use of the 52 K protein as a marker can be proposed.

4. AUTOCRINE CONTROL OF CELL PROLIFERATION BY ESTROGEN REGULATED PROTEIN(S) AND THERAPEUTIC IMPLICATIONS

Previous results support the idea that some of the proteins released into the medium are correlated to, if not responsible for, the regulation of cell growth by estrogens. Estrogens are known to increase the total amount of proteins released into the medium, as well as to induce specifically the 52 K and 160 K proteins. These effects precede the effect of E_2 on cell growth (by 2 days). When the culture media are changed less often, the effect of E_2 on cell growth is much greater, compared to the control, suggesting that the medium is conditioned by factors released by the cells. This observation has also been made by Lippman et al. (21). Conversely, non-steroidal antiestrogens and progestins decrease the production of total proteins released by hormone-dependant cells in culture (6)(14). Several proteins and putative growth factors are secreted by MCF7 cells. In addition to the 52 K and 160 K proteins, the 28 K protein (22) and the pS2 protein (23), obtained secondarily from a cDNA clone, are also regulated by estrogens. The more classical growth factors, TGF α(24) and somatomedine C (25), are secreted by MCF7 cells and may possibly be regulated. Finally, other growth factors of 62 K have been purified from human milk and mammary cancer (26). Without excluding all these candidates, we have recently obtained two series of evidence that the 52 K protein can stimulate the growth of MCF7 cells. The first is indirect and was obtained by studying two antiestrogen-resistant variants (R27 and RTx6) cloned from the wild type MCF7 cells by their ability to grow in 1 μM tamoxifen. When measuring the 4 estrogen-specific responses in these variants and in MCF7 cells, we found that in all three cell lines, tamoxifen was able to increase the number of progesterone receptor sites, and to prevent the production of the pS2 mRNA and of the 160 K secreted protein (Table 3).

Table 3.

EFFECT OF TAMOXIFEN
ON THREE ESTROGEN-RECEPTOR-POSITIVE CELL LINES

	R_p	pS2 mRNA	160 K protein	52 K protein	Cell proliferation
MCF7	+	−	−	−	inhibition
R27 RTx6	+	−	−	+	resistant

Summary of the effects of tamoxifen on 5 estrogen-regulated responses in the antiestrogen-sensitive (MCF7) and resistant (R27 and RTx6) cell lines showing that only the 52 K secreted protein behaves differently in the antiestrogen-resistant variants.

By contrast, the regulation of the 52 K protein was different in MCF7 cells, where it was inhibited by tamoxifen, and in the two resistant variants, where it was stimulated by tamoxifen (27a)(27b). These observations suggest that one way the cells resist antiestrogen is by producing growth factor(s) under antiestrogen stimulation, and that the 52 K protein might be one of these growth factors. The second series of evidence was obtained more directly by assessing the effect of the purified 52 K protein on the growth of quiescent MCF7 cells (Fig. 2).

Figure 2. Basis for studying the mitogenic activity of secreted proteins

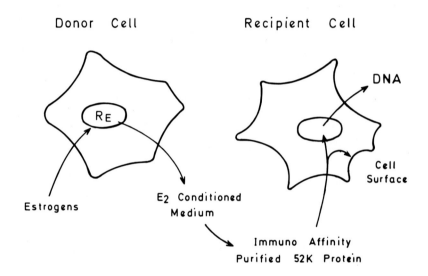

The donor cells are MCF7 cells producing high level of 52 K protein in the medium (20 ng per ug DNA per day) following estradiol stimulation with 10 nM. The recipient cells are MCF7 cells deprived of estrogens for 4 days and growing slowly in 1 % charcoal-treated FCS. These cells produced less 52 K protein. The 52 K protein was purified to homogeneity by two successive affinity columns (Con A and MAb Sepharose) as described (17)(29).

Vignon et al. (28) have previously shown that proteins from serum-free media conditioned by estrogen-stimulated MCF7 cells increase the growth of dormant MCF7 cells, and that the mitogenic activity is retained by Con A Sepharose chromatography and is eluted with the glycoprotein fraction. By contrast, the conditioned media from estrogen-withdrawn MCF7 cells are inactive or inhibitory at high protein concentrations. More recently, using a two-step purification procedure (Con A-Sepharose + immunoaffinity chromatography) we evaluated the biological activity of a homogeneous 52 K protein fraction on the same estrogen-withdrawn MCF7 cells. The dose-dependant stimulation of cell growth, as evaluated by DNA assay, ranged from 120 % to 240 % (Table 4).

Table 4. Mitogenic effects of estradiol, estradiol conditioned medium and purified 52 K protein on MCF7 cells

	Estradiol	E_2 Cond. Medium	52 K Protein
% vs control	290 ± 100^a (10)	530 ± 260^b (7)	170 ± 40^a (11)	170 ± 50^b (7)
% vs E_2 stimulated	100	100	58	32
52 K Protein ng/ml			25-200	2,5-50

The stimulatory effect of these three treatments was evaluated on steroid-deprived MCF7 cells by assaying cellular DNA. The concentration of 52 K protein was determined by IRMA. a and b are from 2 different series of experiment.
(Results are from (28) and Vignon et al (in preparation)).

A mean stimulation of 170 % was obtained in the 7 experiments performed. This stimulation represented 40 % of the effect obtained by estradiol and was observed at 52 K protein concentrations similar to concentrations released into the culture medium (29). We have excluded the possibility that proteins labeled by ^{35}S-methionine or ^{35}S-cysteine contaminate the 52 K protein preparation. The presence of TGFα, Somatomedin C, or pS2 protein in this preparation is therefore very unlikely. Moreover, we recently showed that the 52 K protein could be internalized and processed by the recipient MCF7 cells into smaller forms of 48 and 34 kDa molecular weight (17)(29).

These results suggest that glycoproteins present in the medium act as growth factors, at least partly mediating the mitogenic effect of estrogen on mammary cells. The 52 K protein is among these mitogens, under culture conditions. However, further work is needed to prove that the 52 K protein also functions in vivo as a growth factor since other activities on cancer cells or on adjacent cells (paracrine mechanism) have not been excluded.

5. CONCLUSIONS

The 52,000 dalton glycoprotein, which is secreted under estrogen control in hormone-dependant breast cancer, and constitutively in other RE-negative breast cancer, can now be probed by several monoclonal antibodies. The use of these antibodies has shown that the protein is relatively specific for mammary tumoral epithelial cells. It is not detected at high concentrations in normal mammary epithelial cells, and in other estrogen target tissues. It is therefore a potential tissue marker of hormone dependency in breast cancer and/or high risk mastopathies. However, more extensive clinical studies are required to confirm its practical clinical interest. The identity of the 52 K protein is presently unknown. Its relationship with other estrogen-regulated proteins (a 28 K protein and a 54 K membrane protein (30)), also described in human breast cancer cells, has been excluded in collaboration with several investigators who have kindly provided their specific antibodies. The identification of the 52 K protein as a plasminogen activator was recently excluded after purification (32) and its relevance to the mouse-MMTV-related gp52 is unlikely since it was not detected in mouse mammary tumors and appears to be human-specific. The 52 K protein therefore does not seem to correspond to a known protein previously described in mammary tissues.

Basic studies of the structure and function of the protein indicate that it is a phosphoglycoprotein (18) secreted into the medium, which can be rebound, internalized, and processed by the same MCF7 cells. The protein is also a mitogen when added to recipient cells that produce little 52 K protein. We hypothesize that this in vitro mitogenic activity may also occur in vivo and that the 52 K protein may be an autocrine growth factor produced in larger amounts under estrogen stimulation. Several growth factors have recently been related to oncogenes (32) and it is conceivable that some of them are regulated by steroids and play a role in the promotion of mammary carcinogenesis by estrogens. The study of the structure of the protein, the cloning of its cDNA and gene, and the selection of antibodies able to prevent its mitogenic activity may provide evidence for or against this hypothesis.

ACKNOWLEDGEMENTS

We are grateful to members of our laboratory and of CLIN-MIDY/SANOFI Laboratory (B. Pau) who have contributed to several parts of this work ; to D. Derocq, G. Salazar, C. Rougeot and C. Prébois for technical assistance and to E. Barrié and M. Egéa for their skilfull preparation of the manuscript. We thank Drs M. Lippman, M. Rich, I. Keydar, and the Mason Research Institute, for their gifts of mammary cell lines and Pr P. Chambon for his gift of pS2 cDNA clone.

REFERENCES

1. Banbury Report (1981). "Hormones and Breast Cancer". Pike MC, Siiteri PK, Welsch CW (eds) Cold Spring Harbor Laboratory.
2. McGuire WL (1980). Steroid hormone receptor in breast cancer treatment strategy. In "Recent Progress in Hormone Research", Academic Press, Vol 36, p 135.
3. Lippman ME, Bolan G, Huff K (1976). The effects of estrogens and antiestrogens on hormone responsive human breast cancer in long-term tissue culture. Cancer Res 36:4595.
4. Chalbos D, Vignon F, Keydar I, Rochefort H (1982). Estrogens stimulate cell proliferation and induce secretory proteins in a human breast cancer cell line (T47D). J Clin Endocrin Met 55:276.
5. Darbre P, Yates J, Curtis S, King RJB (1983). Effect of estradiol on human breast cancer cells in culture. Cancer Res 43:349.
6. Vignon F, Bardon S, Chalbos D, Rochefort H (1983). Antiestrogenic effect of R5020, a synthetic progestin in human breast cancer cells in culture. J Clin Endocrin Met 56:1124.
7. DeLarco JE, Todaro GJ (1978). Growth factors from murine sarcoma virus-transformed cells. Proc Natl Acad Sci 75:4001.

8. Westley B, Rochefort H (1980). A secreted glycoprotein induced by estrogen in human breast cancer cell lines. Cell 20:353.

9. Sirbasku DA, Benson RH (1979). Estrogen-inducible growth factors that may act as mediators (estromedins) of estrogen-promoted tumor cell growth. In Sato JH, Ross R (eds): "Hormones and Cell Culture", Cold Spring Harbor Laboratory, Cold Spring Harbor, Vol 6, p 477.

10. Rochefort H, Chalbos D, Capony F, Garcia M, Veith F, Vignon F, Westley B (1984). Effect of estrogen in breast cancer cells in culture : Released proteins and control of cell proliferation. In Gurpide E, Calandra R, Levy C, Soto RJ (eds): "Hormones and Cancer", New York: Alan R Liss Inc, Vol 142, p 37.

11. Adams DJ, Edwards DP, McGuire WL (1983). Estrogen regulation of specific proteins as a mode of hormone action in human breast cancer. In "Biomembranes", Vol 11, p 389.

12. O'Farrell PZ, Goodman HM, O'Farrell PH (1977). High resolution two-dimensional electrophoresis of basic as well as acidic proteins. Cell 12:1133.

13. Vignon F, Terqui M, Westley B, Derocq D, Rochefort H (1980). Effects of plasma estrogen sulfates in mammary cancer cells. Endocrinology 106:1079.

14. Chalbos D, Rochefort H (1984). Dual effects of the progestin R5020 on proteins released by the T47D human breast cancer cells. J Biol Chem 259:1231.

15. Touïtou I, Garcia M, Westley B, Capony F, Rochefort H. High mannose N-glycosylation of the estrogen regulated 52 000-Mr protein secreted by breast cancer cells. Submitted for publication.

16. Garcia M, Capony F, Derocq D, Simon D, Pau B, Rochefort H (1985). Monoclonal antibodies to the estrogen-regulated Mr 52,000 glycoprotein : Characterization and immunodetection in MCF7 cells. Cancer Res 45:709.

17. Capony F, Morisset M, Garcia M, Rochefort H. Purification of the estrogen-regulated 52 K protein secreted by human breast cancer cells. Submitted for publication.

18. Capony F, Capony JP, Chalbos D, Vignon F, Rochefort H. Phosphorylation of the 52 K estrogen regulated protein secreted by MCF7 cells. In preparation.

19. Garcia M, Salazar-Retana G, Richer G, Domergue J, Capony F, Pujol H, Laffargue F, Pau B, Rochefort H (1984). Immunohistochemical detection of the estro-

gen-regulated Mr 52,000 protein in primary breast cancers but not in normal breast and uterus. J Clin Endocrin Met 59:564.

20. Veith FO, Capony F, Garcia M, Chantelard H, Pujol H, Veith F, Zajdela A, Rochefort H (1983). Release of estrogen-induced glycoprotein with a molecular weight of 52,000 by breast cancer cells in primary culture. Cancer Res 43:1861.

21. Jakesz R, Smith CA, Aitken S, Huff K, Schuette W, Shackney S, Lippman M (1984). Influence of cell proliferation and cell cycle phase on expression of estrogen receptor in MCF7 breast cancer cells. Cancer Res 44:619.

22. Edwards DP, Adams DJ, Savage N, McGuire WL (1980). Estrogen-induced synthesis of specific proteins in human breast cancer cells. Biochem Biophys Res Commun 93:804.

23. Chambon P, Dierich A, Gaub MP, Jakowlev S, Jongstra J, Krust A, Lepennec JP, Oudet P, Reudelhuber T (1984). Promoter elements of genes coding for proteins and modulation of transcription by estrogens and progesterone. In Greep O (ed): "Recent Progress in Hormone Research", Academic Press, Vol 40, p 1.

24. Salomon DS, Zwiebel JA, Bano M, Losonczy I, Fehnel P, Kidwell WR (1984). Presence of transforming growth factors in human breast cancer cells. Cancer Res 44:4069.

25. Furlanetto RW, DiCarlo JN (1984). Somatomedin-C receptors and growth effects in human breast cells maintained in long-term tissue culture. Cancer Res 44:2122.

26. Bano M, Salomon DS, Kidwell WR (1985). Purification of a mammary-derived growth factor from human milk and human mammary tumors. J Biol Chem. In press.

27a. Vignon F, Lippman ME, Nawata H, Derocq D, Rochefort H (1984) Induction of two estrogen-responsive proteins by antiestrogens in R27, a tamoxifen resistant clone of MCF7 cells. Cancer Res 44:2084.

27b. Westley B, May FEB, Brown AMC, Krust A, Chambon P, Lippman ME, Rochefort H (1984). Effects of antiestrogens on the estrogen regulated pS2 RNA, 52 kDa and 160 kDa proteins in MCF7 cells and two tamoxifen resistant sublines. J Biol Chem 259: 10030.

28. Vignon F, Derocq D, Chambon M, Rochefort H (1983). Endocrinologie. Les protéines oestrogéno-induites sécrétées par les cellules mammaires cancéreuses humaines MCF7 stimulent leur prolifération. C R Acad Sci (Paris) 296:151.
29. Vignon F, Chambon M, Capony F, Garcia M, Rochefort H The purified estrogen regulated 52,000 daltons protein secreted by MCF7 cells stimulate the growth of those cells. In preparation.
30. Brabon AC, Williams JF, Cardiff RD (1984). A monoclonal antibody to a human breast tumor protein released in response to estrogen. Cancer Res 44: 2704.
31. Massot O, Capony F, Garcia M, Rochefort H (1984). The estrogen-regulated 52 K protein and plasminogen activators released by MCF7 cells are different. Mol Cell Endocrinol 35:167.
32. Heldin CH, Westermark B (1984). Growth factors: Mechanism of action and relation to oncogene. Cell 37:9.

Index